HAPPINESS
Made Crystal Clear!

My Sounds Elevate Your True Joy

DAWN CRYSTAL

outskirts
press

DEDICATION

This is for all those who suffer from unhappiness, and who know the answer is not alcohol or drugs. There are alternative drug-free methods to relieve unhappiness that are safe, effective, and rapid. It takes some guidance and an open mind to obtain the possibilities of these non-traditional methods, including mine.

Table of Contents

FOREWORD

Happiness is clearly a worthwhile goal of living, not the only worthwhile goal, but a truly valuable one. Here we explore some of the barriers to happiness and some approaches to overcoming them.

Some background on my relationship with Dawn Crystal, for whom I became a writing coach and editor:

I "met" Dawn Crystal over the radio, Internet radio station WMAPradio.com, where "WMAP" stands for "World's Most Amazing People," a title for which she qualifies. During an extensive interview with host KC Armstrong, she told how she developed her astonishing techniques for relieving pain, by directing the internal energy of the person being helped. She had previously been interviewed on ABC-TV, *The Today Show, Dr. Oz,* etc. A vivacious and fluent guest, she also hosts her own radio program from Hawaii on alternate Mondays.

Dawn is a pioneer of vocal sound-energy relief of pain and anxiety. She makes pain-relieving, fear-relieving sounds with her voice, a gift she discovered as an adult. She has done this for over 20 years, with individuals or groups.

Years ago a health food store in Hawaii asked her to help "treat" some customers…making her sounds and blowing on their bodies. No medical claims were made. Yet, many people reported feeling much better.

Subsequently, she found that many of her clients reported relief from fear and anxiety. This book goes into that phenomenon, describing her techniques and presenting testimonials to their effectiveness.

She now has a sophisticated web site, <u>DawnCrystalHealing.com</u>. Dawn feels a Higher Power has guided her to go Internet, go global. She started from nothing, "heart-guided," living out of her car for awhile.

Imagine a world free of fear and anxiety. Imagine if sources of pain could be fixed immediately, without drugs. Imagine being fear-free fast and easy. These are among Dawn's missions.

Who does she think should seek help? Anybody. Everybody. People who have tried everything else: holistic, natural, traditional. She's had success with a wide variety of fears, pains, and unhappiness.

Sometimes, she has discovered issues caused by unconscious influences. For example, she found that a client had been sexually abused as a child and didn't remember it.

What to make of all this? The testimonials here are evidence that something beneficial is happening. We know that mind and body are interconnected. Hypnosis and auto-suggestion can produce dramatic changes, including pain and fear relief. Many medical successes are attributed to the "placebo effect," where belief in the likely efficacy of a cure helps produce a cure. Voodoo curses can cause the believers great harm. Human attraction, "animal magnetism," can make us feel better when we are ill or hurting. Faith healers have some surprising results, too.

A study by researchers at Denmark's Aarhus University, reported at neurosciencenews.com on 22 December 2016

[https://neurosciencenews.com/dopamine-genetics-music-5806/],

"Sounds, such as music and noise, are capable of reliably affecting individuals' moods and emotions, possibly by regulating brain dopamine, a neurotransmitter strongly involved in emotional behavior and mood regulation… [it is] highly variable across individuals."

Recently, ideapod.com reported that neuroscientists found that a song, "Weightless," reduced anxiety of a majority of its listeners: [https://ideapod.com/neuroscientists-discover-song-reduces-anxiety-65-now-going-viral-listen/?utm_source=ideapod&utm_medium=email&utm_campaign=broadcast]

Discussing her techniques with Dawn, I found that her description of moving energy throughout the body and overcoming blockages resembled somewhat the techniques I had learned years ago of auto-suggestion, self-hypnosis, in which progressive relaxation is produced by visualizing a warm, relaxing wave traveling through various parts of your body, starting with your feet. I have first-hand knowledge that such techniques worked for me, including relieving occasional tension headaches and facilitating falling asleep.

Those who would like to hear Dawn talk about herself and her techniques are invited to listen to this 25-minute interview done in August 2018, https://www.talkshoe.com/conf/summary/4977560.

I have been pleased to help get Dawn's story into print as her writing advisor and editor. Another kind of personal change occurred: her energy and optimism have been infectious!

Douglas Winslow Cooper, Ph.D.

douglas@tingandi.com

WriteYourBookWithMe.com

Walden, NY 12586, USA

Summer 2019

Acknowledgments

First, and once again, I thank my coach and editor, Douglas Winslow Cooper, Ph.D., without whom this book would never have been written.

My pets – my dog, Hoku (Hawaiian for "star"), and my cats, Stitchy and Blacky – bring me daily joy and peace and deserve my gratitude. I can't imagine my life without them.

DISCLAIMER

The information in this book is not intended to be a replacement or substitute for medical advice. It does not diagnose, treat, or cure medical conditions. Please see a medical professional if you need help with such problems.

Preface

I wrote this book because I wanted everyone to know that there is hope for becoming happier, naturally, fast, easy, and effectively.

You should read this book if you are suffering from frequent unhappiness or you know someone who is, and you or they have tried many different techniques without success to get relief.

As a gift to you, I am including this link to my introductory CD, which is directed toward relieving anxiety and insomnia, which sometimes contribute to unhappiness:

https://drive.google.com/open?id=0B0lQ6PlNYe2AU21mQnpEdTh HekU

"Discover Sound Healing," normally sold for $20. I invite you to experience the soothing sounds channeled through my voice...to realign yourself to your center. In as little as 20 minutes, you should feel peace through your physical body as your stress, anxiety, and worry disappear.

You are also invited to link to my Unlimited Energy program:

Unlimited Energy Program

I am known by many for my healing vocals. I offer my sound healing sessions with a loving heart by phone and in person.

Dawn Crystal

DawnCrystalHealing@gmail.com

Maui, Hawaii

Summer 2019

Prologue: The Hunt for Happiness

We all know how it feels to be happy. We don't know how to generate this feeling consistently. Ideally, we would arrange our lives to be happy all the time, or at least when things aren't going to pot in our vicinity. In the chapters here, we are going to explore various approaches to pursuing happiness:

MONEY: Having a lot of money is no guarantee of being happy, but being in debt can make you feel sad.

LIFE: Life is a gift, unless you are in continuing pain.

FAME: Being famous is fun, until you want some privacy.

LOOKS: Being attractive is a plus, but being beautiful can control your life.

HOMES: You can be too house-proud, too house-poor.

CARS: In Los Angeles they sometimes say you are what you drive. You need to get beyond that.

RELIGION: Some religions bring comfort, fewer bring happiness?

CHILDREN: They are a matter of taste, but they do make your life matter more.

FRIENDS: The more the merrier? If they are for real.

BUSINESS SUCCESS: The satisfaction must be balanced against the sacrifices.

HEALTH: Hard to be happy if you are feeling unwell.

TALENT: It's a pleasure, unless you think it is being unjustly ignored.

LOVE: Makes the world go around. Conquers all. Hard to find. Good to give.

LUCK: If you can read this, you are already a lucky person. Enjoy yourself.

PETS: They ask for so little, and they give us so much.

GRATITUDE: To be happy, make GRATITUDE your ATTITUDE.

Chapter 1

MONEY

"What's the use of happiness? It can't buy you money."
– *Henny Youngman*

HENNY YOUNGMAN'S QUIP turns on its head the familiar adage that money can't buy you happiness, and in so doing emphasizes what we've been told but may find hard to believe: getting a lot of money is not a sure path to being happy, although it often beats being poor, especially being dirt-poor. Once you can stop worrying about the bill-collectors, having money becomes less important than many other things in your life, though some problems can be profitably addressed with a hefty dose of cash.

I grew up in very poor circumstance, a welfare family with six kids, and I was the least cared for. I wore hand-me-down clothes from my older sister, much too big. And I used to have over-sized shoes. I would stick tissue paper in the shoes to keep them from falling off my feet.

My mother went from hand to mouth, with little money, as my dad was not in the picture. I could see that other kids had stuff I did not have, and they would take vacations to places I wished I could go. Disneyworld was a dream! I felt like the Cinderella of the neighborhood.

In second grade, I did not fit in. The kids did not like the way I looked. The after-school activities I wished I could do were ballet and tap-dancing lessons, and the other girls would take these classes, while I watched and wished I could afford to participate.

I shared a room with my younger brother. Two older brothers were in the room next door. They often raised a ruckus. My younger brother would huddle together with me, just as fearful as I was.

I had very few friends; being from a welfare family with little money, I was viewed as somewhat undesirable. Some kind neighbors would invite us kids for meals, feeling sorry for us, but this did not make me feel accepted, especially as my older brothers were notorious for drinking, fighting, and drag racing deep into the night and early morning. I would look out the window at 2 a.m. and see my brothers being chased by cops. My sister was loose, too. My mother seemed never to be home.

After being kept up late up almost every night, I would have to go to school the next morning, poorly dressed, unattractive, a member of a family that most people disrespected. There was little in the way of child protection services in my Chicago in the 1970s, little sympathy or help for me.

At nine, I was being hurt by the kids who were teasing and bullying me because my clothes were weird, and I had buck teeth, from sucking my thumb to pacify myself. I had no supervision as I grew; my over-weight mom was all caught up with herself and her issues and ignored her kids.

I saw that the older kids had paper routes. At age nine, I hoped to buy some clothes that would let me fit in with the other kids and maybe even let me take ballet and tap-dancing lessons.

I got a paper route at nine! I looked older, perhaps because I was stressed. In Chicago, I would collect the money from my route at night. People asked me where my mother was, allowing a kid my age to be out so late. People occasionally would give me extra tips. One lady gave me an extra dollar and sometimes even hot chocolate in the cold weather, but most people did not want to get involved, did not intervene.

My family complained about their lives, but didn't work hard, while taking drugs and alcohol, and my mother would push me to nag my father to get child-support money.

I thought money would make me happy.

My life seems a blur until I reached 14. A neighbor saw what I was going through and asked my mom if I could be taken under her wing, live with her. My mother agreed, and this saved my life, as this woman became like a benevolent aunt. She didn't want anything from this.

During this period, I lost several of my siblings—alcoholics and drug addicts. One brother died from a heroin overdose; another died from complications related to be being beaten severely in a bar. The hardest death was that of my younger brother, a year younger. He and his friends shot up heroin, He died at 16, severely addicted. He would beg to stay with me in my independent apartment, as the home situation was intolerable for him and for me. But he was a compulsive thief, stealing to get drugs. He died a slow, painful death from a staph infection that weakened his heart. These losses made me really think about life. I also think this made me go into law enforcement later. I had a drive to help other people and improve society.

Eventually, I graduated from high school. While there, I started dating a guy in the school band. I had met him when I was 14. Lee was Southern. I liked him a lot, but I did not know what love was like, as I never experienced it from my family. Lee and I got into sex too young, leading to my having a miscarriage at 16. I dated him for nine years, into my early twenties. Frankly, I guess he was using me for sex.

I became pregnant again in my teens, and my mother wanted me to keep it, but Lee did not, so I got an abortion.

I worked as a hostess at IHOP at 16 and was happy that I could buy myself some decent clothes. After graduation from high school, I became a store manager at Dunkin' Donuts.

That relationship with Lee fizzled out in my early 20s.

I was always working. After I graduated from high school, my first job, in a plastics company, in marketing, gave me $25000 per year, a good salary then, but I foolishly got romantically involved with my manager.

I left and joined the Chicago Police Department, passed the tests, made $35000/year and got married to a fellow cop. We bought a condo, and I dressed up. I found myself continuing to chase money and using Xanax to calm me. My husband got hurt and lost his police job; he could not return. I left my job, to take care of him. He was on disability, and I was on unemployment. We then had to sell the condo. My life had fallen apart.

We had a medical lawsuit from which we finally collected a modest amount of money. We lived with his mom in Pennsylvania. Meanwhile, I was taking Xanax and Prozac, my husband on disability, his mother on welfare.

The lawsuit settlement gave us money we didn't know how to handle. We started by getting legal and financial advice, investing it. Then we blew it on an expensive car and a beautiful condo. Sadly, we had no real self-control regarding money, and my husband took to drinking to offset his unhappiness, partly due to his injury. We divorced, split the money, and I opened a couple of businesses, which I was able to make somewhat successful while still depending on Xanax.

I met a man at my tanning salon, a charming, good-looking guy, who liked the way I was bringing in money. He had a job, then lost it, not long after we got married, due to his drinking problem. He was draining me dry. The nest egg was disappearing. He had a bad motorcycle accident, while drunk. That was it…I'd had enough!

The tanning business fizzled, and I was losing money while my condo was losing value. In fact, I went bankrupt. At this low point, I gave away whatever I possessed and moved, severing all ties. I divorced him. He got the house, and I got a one-way ticket to the Hawaiian Islands, following my heart and a magazine ad that said, "Go to the Sun!"

I had given him almost all the stuff we owned, and I headed for Hawaii. Money had not been working for me. I kept only $700 and my jewelry, and landed with two bags of clothes in Hawaii.

Uh, oh, I thought: *why have I done this?*

I got a Rent-a-Wreck that I proceeded live in, and I slowly sold the jewelry to keep myself going and to pay to run the car.

Here, my life changed. I surrendered my heart. Living on McDonald's Dollar Menu, I would go to the beach daily, and then I realized that money was not crucial to happiness: **I had to overcome my anxiety**.

On the beach, my gift of sound-healing came to me. I sang and hummed to calm myself, and people started to stay with me, even gave me tips, as I made my healing sounds in their vicinity. I did some sound-healing. Then I got a job in a jewelry store, part-time, allowing me to get food. I'd bathe by sneaking into hotel resort pools or using the public showers at the beach. I occasionally pawned some more of my jewelry.

Th Hawaiian police wanted vagrants to keep moving, and that included me. They wanted us off the streets. One place they did not push us from was the parking area by the beach, where I went to save on gas money, by not having to move my car so much.

Worried that I was crazy, I was sitting on the beach, humming along, and sounds were coming through my voice, sounds that got stronger and stronger, helping me feel better. I was self-medicating with sound! I did this for hours, stone sober, as I have never been on drugs.

"What are you doing, lady?" a curious beach-goer asked.

"I'm making sounds that help me."

"Can I stay and listen?"

"Yes."

"Your sounds are making me feel better, too."

Some people would sit with me for hours. This was unusual back at that time, as spirituality was generally considered "weird," "voodoo." I went to some health fairs and began collecting tips.

I know why I thought money meant happiness, but I was wrong. I'd been rich, and I'd been poor, and money was not the key to happiness. My Mercedes had not made me merry. The condo had not made me content. Happiness comes from within one's heart.

Instead, my calling as a sound-healer has brought me happiness. Doing what you are created for does bring contentment. It may bring abundance, also, but that is not my goal. I now can be happy whether I have money or not, and that has made me much more stable…better than Prozac, better than Xanax. I have found what I love to do.

It seems I had to go through this trial to reach the state I am in now, and I wouldn't change my now way of living for the world.

Chapter 2

LIFE

"When I went to school, they asked me what I wanted to be when I grew up. I wrote down 'happy.' They told me I didn't understand the assignment, and I told them they didn't understand life." – *John Lennon*

WHEN ASKED WHAT the three most valuable things were to him, a friend of mine wrote, "life, love, and liberty." Life is precious, and we need to be grateful for it. Fortunately for us, the egg and sperm combination that gave rise to our genes produced the unique person we are, rather than another genetic individual, a brother or sister, the one we never became. We must value this opportunity, make the most of it.

As I grew up in a dysfunctional family, my own life revolved around watching them screw up with drink and drugs. This included my three older brothers, and my younger brother got into it, too. I watched them waste away, leaving me numb.

My brother Wayne died from heroin. It didn't move me, but I swore I would not do it.

Brother Bill a few years later killed himself with alcohol.

Younger brother, Gene, not as strong as I, unfortunately followed an older brother into drugs and alcohol. He got an infection that his wasted body couldn't defeat. At age 16! He told me he wished he had done something else with his life. At that point, he was on a breathing machine and couldn't breathe on his own. Sadly, Gene died at 16.

My heart was broken by Gene's death. I decided never to do such a thing, never to touch drugs or booze. I realized life was too precious to waste. That experience with Gene kept me on track. I lacked a mentor, so I became my own mentor.

After these deaths, I really started to find my own way through life.

The police officer job I got was an attempt t give back to other people.

My healing activities have become really the focus of my life, making a difference, while appreciating every moment. Many people find themselves in pain, and I help them escape it.

I recently worked with Jill, who requested a session. She was well off, basically wanted to see what a session was like, hoping to find love, having been married to three different rich men, without finding love. She liked the security of money.

She told me, "I'm in my early 50s, three marriages. Marrying for money seemed a good idea but did not work out. Your story made me want to get to be a happier person, rather one simply chasing money. I know there must be something better. Can you help me? What am I missing? How can I have energy like yours and not be stressed out?"

"Let's get into your body, stabilize your energy. You are not at peace. We are going to clear your energy field. Imagine the bad energy moving out. We will replace it with life-force energy and your higher soul."

I made some of my sounds, clearing her energy.

"Now, how do you feel?"

"Lighter and more peaceful than before."

"Let's see what is making you uneasy. What are your true gifts?"

She had grown up poor. Her parents were not available to her emotionally, which reminded me of my own upbringing. She dreamt of marrying well, marrying wealth.

"We are going to clear some of this unhappy energy from your early years."

She started crying. "I am holding a lot of weight."

"We will clear that. Move that energy out from you." I continued with my sounds. "How do you feel now?"

"Great!"

"Yes. You will no longer be controlled by your inner child. What gifts, what talents do you have?"

"I liked to work with my hands while I was in school. I enjoyed painting but could not make money that way."

"It can be therapeutic for you, and you don't need to start making money with it, though later it might bring you some."

"I'll try that."

I made more of my vocal sounds. She seemed ready to change.

She looked at me and told me, "I'm ready to try my gifts. I see that you are enjoying what you do."

We ended her session with grounding.

She was to email me about our session later. A month later, she wrote that she has dedicated at least an hour a week to create things in a bedroom she has converted into a workroom. She hopes to sell some of these on eBay.

Things were changing for her.

Regardless of our inner child, we must find our true self, which may be a talent or gift, from which we need not make money, though we may. Finding it will give us a sense of satisfaction, especially from sharing it with other people.

Chapter 3

FAME

"Fame doesn't fulfill you. It warms you a bit, but that warmth is temporary." – *Marilyn Monroe*

"I know what it feels like to be hunted….the worship of celebrity…suffocated me….The majority of great actresses meet tragic ends." – *Brigitte Bardot*

Fame is superficial, being what others think about you, rather than what is true…or, at least, rather than what you think is true about yourself.

Fame is fleeting. Last year's celebrity is often this year's has-been. The Latin expression is *sic transit gloria mundi* ("Thus passes worldly glory.") Fame may help you or hurt you. If you are famous for something good, you will receive favored treatment by many. If you are famous for something ill, you will likely be scorned and spurned. Aside from some better or worse treatment, it will boil down to what people think of you, and you really don't want your happiness to be so dependent on other people, many of whom have values you do not yourself treasure.

Fame can be a drag, leading you to seek privacy, with difficulty.

So, fame is fleeting, a mixed bag, superficial, sometimes a drag. What's not to like?

Barbie, her real name, bought my Anti-Aging program and wanted to look like her namesake doll.

She was a new client, and we had a 30-minute session,

"Hi, Barbie, thanks for getting my Anti-Aging program. What do you most want to work on?"

"Actually, I can really relate to you and what I learned about your own life. We both are known world-wide. I am a go-getter, with a fine voice, known by many in the entertainment industry. I've been on the go all my life."

She quickly revealed she had invested in a lot of cosmetic surgery. She had several implants. On our Skype call, I could see some touch-ups had been a bit overdone: lips, nose, chest. Too much, an unreal look. She had tried too hard, emphasizing looks.

"I am tired of this life. I'm 50, and things seem empty, despite my singing career success. In the 1980s, I was in one of those big-hair group bands. Also, I've had some serious romantic relationships. But I've been searching for that ultimate 'aha' moment without finding it."

"You do look very good for your age."

"Thank you. I've had lots of surgeries, for thousands of dollars, and my body does not feel good. I look OK, but it has not brought me happiness. The singing gigs and the plays have gotten me known, but I'm not really famous. I wonder whether I've been wasting my life. I'm not happy, even though I thought I was making the right choices. What do you see for me?"

"Let's look into your energy. Your talent is your voice, but you have gotten side-tracked, emphasizing your looks rather than your singing. And you have not set aside enough time for yourself."

"Right. I have no close relationships, and I feel washed-out."

"We have to clear up the idea that you must over-achieve and become famous to become happy. You need to change direction and pay attention to some parts of yourself that you have neglected."

I did some energy clearing of Barbie with my sounds. I had her imagine a divine light over her head and move energy to it. This was the first time she had energy work done by anyone.

"Barbie, I am going to clear some energy in you that is due to people in your past. I see a future very different from your past, and we are going to cut these old energy cords, these energy connections from your past. I think they are causing you to be depressed."

"Yes, I am depressed."

     HAPPINESS MADE CRYSTAL CLEAR!

She had come from a broken family, with an alcoholic father, and she had sought his love, to no avail. He is dead now. She never heard any praise from him. Her mom did try to help but had her own personal issues; Barbie and her mother had a fairly good relationship, although more of a friendship rather than parent-child love.

I thought I saw her problem. "You have to look into this pattern of overly-serving others, not yourself. First, though, are you willing to forgive your father who did not give you love but did stay and support the family?"

"Yes, I can try. I have had empty relations with men that reflect this problem I had with my dad."

"We are going to clear this hurtful energy built up from the childhood rejection by your dad." I produced more soothing vocalizations.

As I continued working with her, she started to cry, and it was clear she had deep, pent-up emotions. She had been searching for love. A rather long energy-clearing sound session finally led to her stopping crying.

"How are you now? We have cleared a lot of energy from your childhood."

"I have never felt this good in my life! I feel you have filled the void in my life for the first time."

We grounded her energy to the Earth, to help her take a whole new direction in her life. She indicated she was ready for this. "Some things have been coming to my attention lately, and I will take up some new interests. Perhaps photography, for example."

"Good. Your soul wants you to experience more self-love and to connect with nature. Your heart chakra wants you to reunite your childhood self with your present one."

"I've never felt so OK. I see there is nothing more that I have to do in order to be happy. I don't have to do things to make myself happy. I can just be happy. I am so glad I found you, Dawn."

I have not heard again from Barbie, but I believe she is a much happier person now, less concerned about her fame or looks.

I myself had much the same experience in my early life in trying to get my father's love and approval. It led to trying too much to please other people. I forgot myself.

The moral is that we must stop searching outside ourselves for that "aha" moment; the answer is to look within ourselves, instead.

Fame or success will not assure happiness. The go-go spirit will not bring true contentment. We have to slow down, look within, get in touch with our thoughts and feelings. We have to find our true self; then our life will improve radically.

We have to rediscover ourselves, find the right path…and we can.

   HAPPINESS MADE CRYSTAL CLEAR!

Chapter 4

LOOKS

"Beauty does not bring happiness to the one who pos-
sesses it but to the one who loves and admires it." –
Herman Hesse

NOVELIST HESSE WAS only partly right: certainly, those who love and
admire someone/something beautiful can be made happy in so doing.
Our early romantic loves enhanced our appreciation of our beloved
person's beauty. Occasionally, however, we look back and say to ourselves, *what was I thinking?* Love and then marriage for some people
can be like the intake of a large meal, dessert-first.

A mountain of research was recently summarized in the book *Looks:
Why They Matter More than You Ever Imagined,* by Gordon Patzer,

Ph.D. In chapter after chapter, Dr. Patzer demonstrates the effects of "lookism" as documented by a variety of studies in:

- Dating, mating, marriage
- Family dynamics and favoritism
- Treatment in school
- Advancement in the workplace
- Before the law, especially in trials
- Getting elected to public office
- Belief about marriage and career possibilities
- The "dark side": anorexia and bulimia
- The Big Business of beauty

Studies have shown that from birth to death, the more physically attractive people are given preference, and we ourselves, if we are frank with ourselves, know we rather look at a pretty face than a plain one. Yet, being good-looking is not enough. Robert Frost's poem "The Lovely Shall Be Choosers" tells a familiar tale: a beautiful person gets all she asks for, yet the choices were ill-advised, the outcomes unhappy.

Dr. Patzer notes that decades of research studies have confirmed that physical attractiveness plays an important role in all our lives. Perhaps Shakespeare would have amended his own line to read, "The fault, dear Brutus, is not in our stars but in our looks."

The tendency to judge people by their looks is sometimes dubbed "lookism," to take its place with "racism" etc. Unfortunately, this seemingly unfair evaluation can lead to the victims' taking extreme steps to try to correct or offset their perceived appearance flaws.

                    HAPPINESS MADE CRYSTAL CLEAR!

I'll confess, I nearly got killed trying to be beautiful, trying to make my body image perfect.

Growing up, I was the Cinderella, the Ugly Duckling, of my neighborhood, with hand-me-down clothes from my sister. A neighbor girl used to beat me up, pull my hair out. She was six-foot tall, almost two feet taller than I. She simply didn't like my looks. (Frankly, I wasn't crazy about hers, either.)

I stuffed tissue paper in my too-big shoes. I was not "comfortable in my own skin." No parent praised me. No one said I was looking good, being good. I would dream about looking like a Barbie doll.

I was an outcast. Kids shunned me, as I came from a creepy family and looked unattractive. Talk about a broken home! We embarrassed my lower-middle-class neighbors.

For years in school, I had no boyfriends, though my classmates did. I was a bit pudgy, definitely not the way I wanted to look.

Finally, in high school, I had a relationship with a fellow in a band, perhaps on the strength of my big disco-era hairdo. He had lots of other girls looking at him, too, as he was a drummer on stage.

I was desperate to improve my looks. I started to work and saved money, putting it aside, and I thought I'd use my credit card to get something I long wanted: plastic surgery. The advertisements' before/after pictures were miraculous.

I made an appointment with a plastic surgeon. I wanted my body made better, with liposuction throughout. I drove myself there and back. The surgery seemed to go well. At home, I felt somewhat off, then developed dizziness, which became shock. I was very thirsty. From the liposuction I had lost too much fluid. I was dangerously dehydrated. My regular doctor, a G.P., could not really help me, even over a few months, a hellish period during which water could not re-hydrate me, as I could not absorb it. My skin was wrinkled, and I looked bad. Amazingly, areas had fat that should not have had any. Fat ankles? Fat elbows?

This was a disaster. It took years for my body to get back to near-normal, and even so, I had scars. I had a nose-job, to remove a bump on my nose. I was in pain afterward. I couldn't breathe from one nostril. I had to have the repair itself repaired years later.

I am not going to detail all the surgeries I had, but they were many too many. I kept hoping that surgery would make me look like Barbie, of Barbie doll fame. I came to realize that after all those years trying to make myself look good, and the thousands of dollars I spent, that I would have done better to leave my body unchanged and get counselling instead.

Now that I am adult, I know this has happened to lots of young people, especially young women. I look at this as a learning experience, knowing that changing my looks was not the key to happiness. Changing my thoughts was crucial.

As my sound therapy helped relieve my traumas, I began to feel joy, which made me more attractive than the unhappy Dawn Crystal. I beautified myself from inside out.

Studies show that men tend to judge women's looks by their weight, and women tend to judge men by their height. Knowing that weight is so important to romantic opportunities, as well as to health, many of my female clients come to me for weight loss.

     HAPPINESS MADE CRYSTAL CLEAR!

I worked with a client, call her "Nicole," who bought my recorded weight-loss program that I did with a telesummit.

I offered a 30-minute telephone session to accelerate weight loss.

"I bought your program. I have been heavy all my life. I'm 40 pounds overweight. Let's get the weight off."

She was eager, a bit impatient. I scanned her energy. She is married, with kids, but her husband was not living with them; they were separated, having gotten on each other's nerves.

"Does he kind of drain you?" I asked Nicole.

"Yes."

"Your energy system seems blocked, stagnated. As though you have been unhappy for years."

"True. For financial reasons we have lived apart for decades." She had once been an independent woman. She had begun to feel trapped. I could also sense her metabolism was slow.

"How were you treated as a child?"

"I was adopted, and I was sad about that. We lived near my biological parents, but I felt I had been passed along."

"You did not feel wanted. Even in the womb you sensed your mother was going to be giving you up once you were born. You were aware of that, even in the womb. We need to get your energy going. You are stuck in your marriage, in your life, and lacking unconditional love."

I started making my therapeutic sounds. "Move your energy over your head." I had her energy move through her body. Then, I had her sit down.

"Breathe more deeply, as I move energy through your body. How are you feeling?"

"I'm feeling better."

Her neck and shoulders were tight. I made a different set of sounds. "Is that better now?"

"Yes, I have had excruciating pain there."

"Imagine you are in your mother's womb, not wanted. You did not have the acceptance and love your sought."

"Yes, I feel that. I was not getting love."

"Your birth mother was unsure and tentative and did not give you love from the start."

"I can picture that." She stared crying, her feelings coming up, deep feelings rising from her abdominal area.

A bit later, I asked, "How are you feeling now, Nicole?"

"Something is happening, some movement in my stomach."

We continued the session, and then I concluded it.

I asked her, again, "How are you feeling?"

"Invigorated, with more energy in my body."

"Yes, I have sped up your metabolism, targeting your thyroid. Do you see how your blocked energy contributed to your being overweight?"

"Yes. I feel it."

"You need to make some changes. You need to feel unconditional love. Tell yourself that you love yourself and are worthy of being loved."

She seemed happier, "I feel great! My unconscious pattern has caused me to gain weight."

"You'll change your eating and movement patterns, too."

"Thanks, Dawn, for this very positive session."

Chapter 5

HOMES

"A house is made of walls and beams;
A home is built with love and dreams." – *Anonymous*

A FRIEND OF a friend came to the U.S. from a foreign country where a person's importance was largely measured by the grandeur of his house and grounds. After some years here in the U.S., he succeeded in buying the most expensive place he could barely afford, became "house-poor," which limited his options, and he was eventually divorced by his wife, who ended up with the "mansion." We mustn't measure ourselves or others so superficially, and we certainly should not imagine that a baronial estate will make us happy.

On my own journey, before I went through my spiritual awakening, I had many homes. My first was a beautiful condo I bought by myself in Chicago when I was single and a police officer.

I got married to a fellow officer, and we decided the condo was too small, so we purchased another lovely place, a four-bedroom, newly renovated.

After he lost his eyesight and his career, we were forced to move to live near his mom, in Pennsylvania, living in temporary housing until his disability settlement came in. When it did, we bought a penthouse condo over-looking scenic Lake Erie. Gorgeous! Lavish! I thought we had arrived! But then I found myself worrying about paying the bills, and I never truly enjoyed being there. Living there for three years, we ended up getting divorced.

The man who became my second husband moved into that Lake Erie place. That marriage failed too. When this second marriage failed, we split the proceeds of selling the house. I bought a new four-bedroom home, which I designed from the ground up. Lovely, but I was solitary there, very depressed. It was OK, but not the source of true happiness.

Clearly, having a nice house or not having one did not control my happiness. I was confused, nearly suicidal. I realized my happiness was not in my housing.

I took off for the Sun, heading to Hawaii on a one-way ticket, letting my house go to foreclosure. Stuff was not the key to my happiness. Leaving my "stuff" behind helped free me, even as I became a homeless "street person," living out of my Rent-A-Wreck for six months…and then my gift of sound-healing came to me.

God gave me my gift, and this taught me that my route to happiness is not in gaining material things, but in living in harmony with myself and my calling to help others.

A new client, Mildred, found me a few months ago. We started with a 30-minute session.

"Hi, Mildred, you bought my abundance program. I'll work on that or something else. What would you like to work on today?"

"My husband and I work in real estate. We have a house in the Hamptons, another in Mexico, another in Spain, and another in Tahiti. I'm exhausted keeping them up. I feel like I'm the cleaning lady. The Hamptons are pretty but cold in the winter. They are beautiful, but maintenance is a pain. I grew up overseas in Czechoslovakia, in a business family. We were well off. I grew up with a gold spoon in my mouth.

"Let's work on happiness. I need to unwind. I've got all I wanted, but I cannot relax. I thought you could help me. Something about you seemed to be what I need."

"Looking at your energy, Mildred, I can see it is tied up in a knot. You have had a lot of responsibility for others and for these possessions."

"I do tend to over-give to others. "

"You have forgotten about the need for self-care, about giving to yourself."

"I run the houses, and my husband just likes to travel. I see now that we should start down-sizing, otherwise we are tied to these houses."

                                    HAPPINESS MADE CRYSTAL CLEAR!

"Let's relax you and do some clearing." I made my sounds and had her picture a Divine Light above her head, into which she was to project anything that was not working well for her.

She noted she was taking lots of herbal supplements. They had not cured her tension.

"Let's release some energy. Take deep breaths…. How are you feeling?"

Her breathing had slowed, and she looked less tense.

Her father had been wealthy but not available emotionally to her. Her mother was vain, not available either. Nor did her younger brother really connect with her. She lacked favorable attention. She wanted approval, but she got little or none.

I asked her, "Would you like to change now? Are you ready to downsize? Would you be happier with two properties, not four?"

"That sounds good to me!"

We cleared some of that energy from her childhood. She was ready for the change. She told me, "I can tell you are right. I need to make a change, to drop some of these properties, to get over the sense I have to be responsible for other people."

We did more clearing. She cried, a clear sign of emotional release. I had her breathe more regularly.

"Would you like to clear the belief that you must concentrate on pleasing your husband?'

"I do need to clear that belief." Doing this, she seemed relieved.

We worked a few extra minutes.

"Oh, my God, you are the first healer with whom I feel I've had a breakthrough. I no longer feel I must work to keep everything together. My mission needs to be to take better care of myself. I am releasing the tension from my childhood." She was quite right.

After the session ended with a grounding, I asked her to write to me in a month or so about how she is doing.

"I'm going to discuss with my husband about dropping some of our properties. Thank you for this break-through."

I have not heard from her, but I think she is likely to be doing well.

The moral of that story is that our belief systems often come from our families and the media, such as thinking we must have more to be happy. That "more" includes property, homes...and you can see that this did not bring her happiness, but in fact bogged her down. Mildred realized that less stuff could mean more happiness. "Less is more."

Life is about enjoying what is here now. Be wary of the risk of having too much, of being tied down and distracted with "stuff."

 HAPPINESS MADE CRYSTAL CLEAR!

Chapter 6

CARS

"The cars we drive say a lot about us."
– Alexandra Paul

IT HAS BEEN said that in California, "you are what you drive." Such is also the message in this quote from actress Alexandra Paul. To what extent is this true? Can a Cadillac, a Mercedes, or even a Porsche bring us happiness?

Surely, beautiful things bring pleasure, which can contribute to happiness. Things that do well what they are designed to do are beautiful in achieving their purposes.

Having a car that impresses others, on the other hand, is risky. If you are in the dating game, you may attract someone quite superficial, someone who values your possessions and not you. You may make yourself a target of someone who would steal your car or would deface it out of envy. Later in life, you may make your neighbors jealous or, if your car is old and dirty (as some of mine have been), you may be treated poorly for parking an eyesore in a conspicuous place.

A sports car may make you prone to taking chances on the road, may be more powerful or difficult for you to handle.

A sensible, economical, environmentally-friendly vehicle can add to your happiness legitimately.

Dr. "Dennis," a doctor of chiropractic I see regularly for fine-tuning, does a good job on my body, which sometimes wears down a bit due to my work with other people's energy. He lives on one of the islands here in Hawaii. He is not just a doctor but also a friend.

In his early 60s, Dr. D. is still single. Brilliant. Not attractive. I respect his ability, but he needs to be more fluffed and buffed for dating. He needs some dressing advice, like not keeping a towel around his neck to absorb sweat! His office needs dusting, and the wallpaper is "Brady-bunch" era, rather old.

I was initially unimpressed by this superficial stuff, but he came to impress me with his skills.

During a typical appointment, we chit-chat about his life, and as a single man, he wishes to have some romantic activity. He is viewed as a "mad scientist" or "Dr. Computer" and, frankly, he needs wardrobe-reconstruction.

                                    HAPPINESS MADE CRYSTAL CLEAR!

Dating different women on the island, he has not found anyone who sticks. It depresses him, and I work to help him become more upbeat.

One of his problems was his car, almost something rescued from a junkyard, a near-wreck given in exchange for his work, by a cashless patient. Unimpressive. When Dr. D. went on dates, he was so embarrassed by his car, he would avoid bringing it to the date, parking it blocks away. Rather than using it to get his date to the restaurant, he'd meet her there instead.

Hawaii is hilly, and his car often could not make it up the hills. He and I would meet in a lower area to get around this problem or I'd drive to his office. Not long ago, he told me he was amassing cash to get a better car for dating.

Recently, I was with him and saw he had a relatively new car. Somehow, he had bought himself an upgrade, a better car. At first, he was quite a bit happier, more confident. He had the car washed and vacuumed inside…a real automotive transformation!

I was diplomatic about how much better this car was than his prior car. Yes, and washing it was a definite plus, a good thing.

He told me, "I took it to a car wash. First time. I used to just wait for the rain to come. Then I went on a date, and I felt more confident than before."

It was not a cure-all; they did not get engaged after few dates, so he felt slightly disrespected. In fact, they broke up.

I was reluctant to tell him that his next effort would have to be toward personal hygiene. He needs more washing and buffing, just as the car did.

I gave him the hint.

I added, "When you go out, you might wear some contact lenses, and do what you did with your car for your own appearance and get a better-looking outfit."

You see, Dr. D. did not find happiness from his first rust-bucket, but the second car, a "chick-magnet," seemed to him likely to help. Unfortunately, what he really needed was to spiff up his own appearance, I told him.

We'll see what happens.

Chapter 7

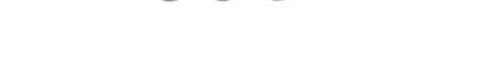

RELIGION

"Happy is the soul that has been awed by a view of
God's majesty." – *A. W. Pink*

IT IS NOT generally the goal of religion to bring happiness, but some faiths do, and many people have found happiness, contentment, comfort in the religion of their choice.

If there is a Creator, and I believe there is, it seems He would design a benevolent world for us. We would not likely understand it fully, and what seems bad to us might have an important purpose. A world with life, love, and liberty would have the possibility of happiness and virtue along with the risks of sadness and evil. Religion can make this situation more acceptable to our thinking, thus promote our happiness.

I worked with David yesterday. His significant other is his long-time love. She has been following my work for years, and I've done a little over-the-phone work with her, some free mini-healings.

She bought him a sound-session package. This generous gift from Lynn to David was my Soul Embodiment Program, which includes a 30-minute session, which he called me for:

"David, how did you find me?"

"Through my girlfriend, Lynn."

He was born into a family of Jehovah's Witnesses, and their beliefs shaped his early life. He felt they boxed him in, but sheltered him, too. He did not truly choose his religion, but it was given to him, as happens with many people. David was angry about being constrained by religion, feeling that he could not give what skills he had to the world.

He became addicted to liquor for a while, became an alcoholic. Fortunately, he had an epiphany, "saw the light," a major change. He met Lynn, and they have been together for many years. His heavy drinking was cured. He departed from Wall Street and became a manager of RV park. He and I both shared that kind of journey, from rich to poor to contentment. Lynn helped him with that. He simplified his life, calmed himself down, and she let him spend time working on himself.

"Now, I'm ready to step it up a notch, to help motivate other people to find themselves, as I have. "

"OK, you left the Witnesses, yet you still believe in God, in a more flexible, intimate way."

We worked on getting him clear, to prepare him to help others. He wanted an abundance orientation. His family had been poor, barely scraping by, which was very limiting.

"Clear the stagnant energy by imagining it to move through your body and out the top of you head. Imagine a light above you absorbing all this energy."

I moved my tones to higher frequencies, as David's energy was being moved upward from his body.

"How do you feel?"

"Oh, my God, I feel so much better! I had been listening to your Soul Embodiment program every day. I was sold on your work even before Lynn bought me this extra session."

"You are ready to take off like an eagle. Now is a good time to see what you can do!"

"I have a coaching certification."

"Good. Credentials are often of use, David."

The first clearing I did for him was to expel the inherited negative energy. We cleared those old voices from his childhood. I had him breathe in a controlled fashion. He had taken on too much of that restrictive religion as a child. Then we moved to Abundance clearing, a silent clearing technique, for a few minutes.

"Think about the things that are not working for you toward gaining abundance"

Meanwhile, I was using my voice, moving energy, clearing his unconscious mind.

"Breathe more deeply. We are getting rid of the unconscious stress that comes from the old stuff. How do you feel?"

"This session is priceless. I'm on a cloud, more inspired. You've cleared my mind, and I am breathing more effectively. I have traction and no longer feel stuck. I am going to look for new things to do to contribute to the world."

Incidentally, he has resumed reading the *Bible*, which I do also.

"David, I think you should journal. We tend to complain about the negative. Instead, list what it is you want. Make an exit plan to escape from your current problems."

"I'll do that. I'm too focused on what I don't have. I would like to make more money."

"Let's seal this session with a special set of sounds. The sounds can be expected to work for days. We'll start from your feet and move your energy. Now, take another deep breath. How do you feel?"

"Oh, my gosh, I do feel like a new person. I will have to have another session with you. I think your humble beginnings connect with my own story, as though our lives were in parallel."

"Thank you, David."

"I'll be calling you in a month to tell you how things have gone."

David story is like mine. I grew up in the Catholic religion, which I found limiting. I did not choose it, it had chosen me, all the way to my Confirmation. My brother and I would head to church, grab a bulletin, skip the service, then douse ourselves with some holy water and return home as though we had gone through Mass. The bulletin was the "evidence."

Over the years, while I left formal religion, I went through homelessness and serious soul-searching, and I have ended up feeling a connection with a Holy Spirit, comforted by reading the Bible for myself. Religion, formal or informal, has a valuable place in the lives of many.

Chapter 8

CHILDREN

"I have learned that raising children is the single most difficult thing in the world to do. It takes hard work, love, luck, and a lot of energy, and it is the most re-warding experience you can ever have." – *Janet Reno*

MANY PARENTS WOULD agree with this quotation from former U.S. Attorney General Janet Reno, yet nearly one in five American women now exit their childbearing years without having a child, whereas it was one in ten in the 1970s. The more education these women have, the fewer children. I myself have not had a child, nor has my editor, though he has been a step-father to a son from age two on, and he found it very satisfying.

One study (reported by Katherine Dorsett, CNN, 24 May 2011) found "parents of all types and all socioeconomic levels in the United States report more symptoms of depression and emotional distress than their childless adult counterparts (Robin Simon, Wake Forest University). Marital satisfaction decreases after the birth of the first child and thereafter. Harvard psychologist Daniel Gilbert is quoted to the effect that children provide many things "but an increase in daily happiness is probably not among them." Part of this may be the expense, estimated as over $200,000 to raise a child in the U.S. to age 17.

And yet, and yet. My editor has had a truly happy and fulfilling calling as a step-parent, and now that their home is childless, he wishes there were another offspring still in the house. However, the investment in bringing up another child was one they did not make, so it is only their own decisions that have left them with an empty nest. At least the son and daughter-in-law occasionally visit. Supporting this, the Dorsett article notes that a recent study worldwide showed that the more children parents over 40 had, the happier they were.

Some people think they need to have children to be happy. Others think they are unhappy because of the children they have.

My pets are my children. They don't talk back. They are happy, non-rebellious, unconditionally loving, no matter what I do. I love them, too.

I recently worked with Marge, also living Hawaii. For fifteen years we've worked together with my sessions. Now in her thirties, she had come here, as I had, on a spiritual journey. I semi-seriously say that she has an old soul in a young body.

We work to clear the damage from her childhood traumas. Marge had been sexually abused by a "friend of the family" in her youth. She has an understandable lack of trust, especially of men.

In one of our sessions, she revealed she very much wanted to be a mother. She grew up having a step-father, not much of a real father figure. She was looking for a surrogate father in the men she dated.

I realized she needed guidance. I asked her what goals she had, what her soul is telling her to do.

In one session, she said, "I want to be a mom. My friends are all moms. I'm not even in a relationship."

Her relationships with men were clearly searches for fathers to take care of her. Often, once they realized what she sought, the men shied away. A half-dozen affairs failed. Marge wondered why.

I was clearing out the layers of trauma from these failed relationships. She would get better, then have a relationship, get in trouble, and contact me to help her escape.

Marge still hopes to be a mother; however, she no longer thinks she must have a child to be happy. Rather, she must first work on her own issues.

I told her, "If the Universe wants you to have a child, Marge, it will happen. Don't force it."

She has followed this advice, and her current romance is going much better.

Another lady, Betty, contacted me after a telesummit; she requested an anti-aging session, but she had different needs that soon became evident; this often happens in these interactions.

     HAPPINESS MADE CRYSTAL CLEAR!

Betty grew up in a lower-middle-class family. Besides the usual money worries, she had a lot of abuse as a child from loveless parents.

As she grew up, being good-looking, she had many men interested in her, and she had three marriages, ending up with a total of eight kids.

She thought, as she grew up, that having kids would bring her happiness, but life did not turn out that way, and the children were not the security blankets she had sought. When the marriages split, the child support was not enough to offset the stress from the variety of concerns these children raised.

Her third marriage was ready for divorce, and she called me.

"I've got eight kids. I thought they would be my happiness. They were joys as little kids, but now that they are older, they are not behaving the way I'd like."

I gave Betty my opinion, "You seem to be having these children for security and for healing your old wounds, right?"

"Yes, no one has said that to me before, but I think you are quite right."

We worked during few sessions to clear her childhood wounds and relieve her sadness. She was nearly numb to start, then became able to feel her true feelings.

The kids had become problems as teenagers. Even though she was well off financially after the divorces, she was unhappy.

What did she want? She hoped to gain enough confidence to be able to become independent. Beyond that, she needed to feel worthy of happiness.

After two sessions, she thanked me and said she felt better. She no longer felt that she would need to look for a fourth husband, nor produce more babies.

A month later, she contacted me. Things had improved. The divorce she wanted was going through without trouble. She thanked me again for the sessions.

Betty is going to live on her own, not look for another man, but go back to school or start a hobby. She certainly seems to have improved her situation.

The bottom line: both healing-session clients thought that children would be the key to happiness. The real key was to heal the wounds from their childhoods. With their permissions, I helped clear for them these toxic energy reserves. I was able to clear the areas that needed to be cleared: for Marge, the lack of a father, and for Betty, the inability to feel emotions. The shifts occurred for these women in a short period of time. They are both now better able to handle the changes that will come into their lives.

Chapter 9

FRIENDS

"Outside of a dog, a book is man's best friend. Inside of a dog, it's too dark to read." – *Groucho Marx*

"If you want a friend in Washington, D.C., get a dog." – Sometimes attributed to President *Harry S. Truman.*

"A friend is one who walks in when the rest of the world walks out." – *Walter Winchell*

FRIENDS ARE IMPORTANT and, for some people, rare. Will they bring you happiness?

Friends certainly seem of value. When you are in need, they should be helpful, as goes the adage, "A friend in need is a friend indeed." If they walk the walk on your behalf, not just talk the talk, then we might re-write the adage as, "A friend, when you are in need, is a friend in deed." Skeptics would say that the sentence could refer to the behavior of a needy friend of ours who pretends to more friendly to assure our aid. But we try to be skeptical only rarely.

Some people are psychologically wired to enjoy, and perhaps need, friends more than others, and if you are this way, then invest in making friends: help, keep in touch, do things together, encourage them. Know, however, that they may not be available or willing when you want help. Self-reliance is always a plus.

Before you marry, be friends with your intended spouse. When you have children, you will need to guide them, to be their parent when they are young, but you can hope to be friends with them when they are grown up. Train them to be likable, if you can.

At the web site happify.com, Jennifer Abbasi has posted her fine article, "Why Friends Make Us Happier, Healthier People," [https://www.happify.com/hd/why-friends-make-us-happier/] making the following points:

The Happiest People Are the Most Social: She credits researchers Ed Diener and Martin Seligman (a widely respected author and long-time investigator of happiness influencers) who compared the happiest to the least happy people and found that the more social people were, the happier.

Happiness Is Contagious: Abbasi cites a Harvard University study of 5000 people over a period of 20 years that found that having a happy friend made you 15% more likely to be happy in that year; an unhappy friend lowered your probability of happiness by 7% in that year.

Friends Cut the Small Talk – and that Makes Us Happy: People who tend to be happy also tend to have more substantive talks with friends than just small talk.

We Turn to Friends When We Are Stressed: This has been found to be especially true for women.

Our Friends Help Us Feel Optimistic: Optimism supports happiness and friendships support optimism…if you pick supportive, upbeat friends.

Friendships Improve Our Health: Social support helps us keep up with our health care, including exercise; with social support, we lose our memory half as fast as those without social support; we are less prone to depression and suicide; we are less likely to have heart problems.

Our Friends Help Us Live Longer: "A review of 148 studies found that people with stronger social relationships have a 50% lower risk of mortality." Of course, we are all going to die someday, but having friends slows that down.

In growing up, I had few friends. I was a misfit in hand-me-down clothes, with buck teeth from sucking my thumb, a homely outcast. My only friends when growing up were a hamster named "Fluffy" (Mom would not let me have a dog), and I tended to connect with nature outdoors.

After my failed marriages, I was living as a hermit, homeless. It was hard for me to trust anybody, for even my school teachers had been mean to me when I was young.

Today, I have worked on myself and healed myself, with loving relationships going beyond pets. The homeless period I got over, and I became more trusting of people, which has made me a better healer.

There are good people on this planet, I came to realize, and I became more and more trusting, having a sixth sense that determined who would be beneficial for me.

The few friends I have now are good friends. My clients are friends to a degree, too. My trust in others has increased.

I still love animals, like my beloved dog Hoku and my nearly half-dozen cats. Even having just a few people you can trust can add great value to your life.

Life surprises us. It is not clear I would have developed my healing gift if I had been distracted by having many friends before the gift came to me. So, this life course has actually worked out for me. The need to heal myself eventually gave me the ability to heal others, too.

A client I worked with for years, "Marcie," had been sexually molested as a child. This caused wounds that needed healing. We started her clearing when she was in her early thirties. She needed to regain her personal power. Fortunately, she is a spiritual person, which attracted us to each other.

In her relationships with men, she was sexually exploited. She chose the wrong kind of men, who then took advantage of her. She needed to heal herself to choose better and interact more suitably. She was too clingy, having not had a father from a young age on. (She used the men as father figures, which made having sex a strange

　　　　　　　　　　HAPPINESS MADE CRYSTAL CLEAR!

situation.) She was dependent, and the men, sensing weakness, treated her badly.

She needed to understand that she did not need other people to be happy, that she is a complete person in herself. With this understanding, she is now attracting true friends who are treating her better, and she is not nearly so dependent. This is quite an evolution.

So, friends are a nice plus, but we must not need them for our happiness. When you don't need them, when you appreciate them and they appreciate you, even having a few solid relationships is better than having a multitude of poor ones. Now, Marcie is planning to marry soon a man who is treating her much better than those she had been with before.

My observation from working with myself and with others is that friends are important, but first we have to get to know ourselves, and accept ourselves, to be able to have true friendships. Else, the relationships tend to be exploitive.

Friendships that are mutual and equitable can contribute to our happiness meaningfully, over the long-term, and some can even last a lifetime.

Chapter 10

Business Success

"A career is wonderful, but you can't curl up with it
on a cold night." – *Marilyn Monroe*

"We make a living by what we get, but we make a life
by what we give." – *Winston Churchill*

ACHIEVING OUR GOALS brings us pleasure. If our goals are suitable, achieving them also gives us a life we enjoy, and we are happy. It is prudent and proper to make enough money for yourself and your family and to do some charitable things as well. More than that may not be needed,

Marilyn Monroe's quip reminds us that warm relationships can be more valuable than money and possessions, whether you are curling up with a lover or a pet.

Winston Churchill emphasized that giving brings more satisfaction, builds a life, more valuable than acquiring things.

In his *12 Truths for Life*, psychologist-philosopher Dr. Jordan B. Peterson maintains that happiness results from having responsibility and fulfilling it. Some of that can be achieved in business, but more often it is achieved in our family and community interactions and our efforts to alleviate suffering.

It has been said that no one puts on his tombstone, "I wish I had spent more time at the office."

For most of my life, I daydreamed about what it would be like to have money. As a child, I wanted to be in the special classes, like ballet and tap dancing, but I couldn't afford it. At nine, I got that paper route to get money and become happy by buying whatever I wanted. I did it a couple of years, and it did help by allowing me to get some better clothes. I kept alert for other business opportunities. I hoped money would bring happiness. Lack of money can certainly bring unhappiness.

As a teen, I had other jobs, like waitressing, and I paid for my own things. Years after graduating from high school, I went into law enforcement and eventually started my own businesses, from the ground up, without training. I was determined. I just knew this would relieve my pain. It did help to have more money, but it wasn't everything. My marriage failed; it became clear that money wasn't enough. I gave my stuff away and moved to Hawaii.

So, my belief that business success would bring happiness was mistaken. I could not even enjoy my expensive house and car. Further, I worried about paying for them.

Moving to Maui without possessions, I've found happiness here. My healing business has brought me prosperity but that does not seem the key; rather, it is that I am helping the people I work with. I am now doing what I should have been doing all along.

Being globally known is fun; the income is not the major part of the satisfaction I get. I learned that happiness does not come from business success, but from a sense of giving value to others.

One of my recent clients who bought my Abundance program was already very well off. She was a lovely woman, with a successful husband, selling artistic figurines worldwide. Some successful people, like Susan, want more success. She and her husband have two homes, one in Hawaii. They are trying to downsize. She would like her husband to spend more time with her.

"Susan, how can I help you?"

"We'd like more, but my husband is working himself ragged. We cannot seem to raise our income. I want us to become more effective at making enough money to have personal time for ourselves."

"Susan, would your husband like to join us?"

"No, he is religious, but he's not into what you and I are doing."

"Tell me about your childhood."

"My mom never trusted my father, who had cheated on her with other women. I had trust issues, too."

"We are going to clear that."

"Good, because I find myself micro-managing the business and worrying about money, even though we have so much."

					HAPPINESS MADE CRYSTAL CLEAR!

"We need to help you find guidance to get your childhood self out of your way. We have to move that old energy from you and get you to trust in a Higher Power, which will help you in your business and with your husband. Take a step back and think about what you should be doing, perhaps outside of business. You have more to offer to the world. What are your gifts?"

"I have no idea."

We did some clearing of the belief systems that she had picked up from family and husband. We worked to get her own energy to be in control.

"Take a few deep breaths. How do you feel?"

"Much more relaxed."

"Good. Since your husband is not into this, you can be an example to him, by getting your own life in spiritual control. You can be a rock, a stable center for him, to help him become more trusting."

"I cannot believe you are telling me this. I do need to trust others more."

"You will save much energy by ridding yourself of that nervous fear, which itself attracts fear and negativity from others."

"My God, I feel so much better! "

I worked with her to dispel her fears. She was not to worry about some-day being homeless, without money. I reassured her that such things can be handled.

"You will never be homeless! Relax! Try to work less and enjoy your life more. Your spiritual path will bring you to trust other people and other creatures on the planet. I am giving you an energy flow to invigorate you."

She left our conversation on a journey to get more spiritual abundance in her life She said she felt calmer and clearer and steadier than she felt at the start.

"I will make an effort to trust our workers and others more. I'd like another session with you. I feel energized."

She did contact me a month later. Her life had been changing. Her husband was responding to her own change and being more trusting. They planned to take a vacation that they had not done before and to take vacations every three months, to ease up, letting others help more with the business. She thanked me for the big changes in her life. I have not heard from her since, but I am confident her life has improved.

From my own life and from working with others, I understand it is great to be prosperous, but we need more: we need to get in touch with our Higher Self. We have this with us always. We have to return to our true selves. This source of energy knows that all is OK. It can energize you to produce changes in your life that no longer will keep you from what you deserve.

Trust is key. Also, we need downtime, and we need to expend some of our efforts to help others.

Chapter 11

HEALTH

"Happiness is good health and a bad memory." – *Dr. Albert Schweitzer*

"Happiness is good health and a bad memory." – *Ingrid Bergman*

THEOLOGIAN-HUMANITARIAN **DR. SCHWEITZER** and drop-dead-gorgeous film actress Ingrid Bergman agreed on this, and perhaps only on this.

Poor health is a drag, and good health is a blessing, so one should invest in keeping well, if one can.

But what if you cannot? We know very well a woman who has been bedridden for 24 years, quadriplegic and on a ventilator for the last 14 of them, due to multiple sclerosis. Somehow, she has found a way to enjoy what she can, to thank those who help her, to express her love to many. She is admirable, but not unique, as many others have overcome illness and disability to find happiness.

We appreciate good health, yet we must prepare for periods of illness and, if we are lucky enough to live to be elderly, we must prepare for a loss of abilities we took for granted. We should enjoy good health while we have it.

Here's a link to a session done concerning body rejuvenation:

https://live.youwealthrevolution.com/popular.php#replay-dawn-crystal.

Finding happiness in having a "bad memory" amuses. Yes, we are well advised to forget bad times and old grudges. Ironically, the aging process does some of this for us automatically. Recent statistics on dementia indicated that by age 65, 1 in 10 Americans suffer from this loss of memory, and by age 85, 1 in 3 do. This seems sad, but perhaps those so affected live in a happier state of mind than we realize.

Growing up, my whole life seemed to be dealing with medical issues. I was awkward, the class "ugly duckling," and I envied those good-looking girls. Part of the problem was my sister's over-sized hand-me-downs I was wearing in school.

In my teens, I tried various surgeries that were mistaken. The worse of these was such that my body shut down after a whole-body liposuction. I tried to look like a Barbie doll. Sadly, I had little money and got the surgery at a cut-rate, using my credit card that I maxed out as a teenager. The surgery was a failure, my body was damaged and bandaged up, with drains attached. I looked like a character from a horror film. My body went into shock. I kept drinking water, but

     HAPPINESS MADE CRYSTAL CLEAR!

my body could not process it. I was nearly bedridden, and I could not work.

I understood this was a big mistake. I had to learn to live with the body I was given, and not risk my health. My health was much more important than looking good.

I had been athletic, and that helped pull me through. I realized that health was crucial to me. That shift changed my life. I no longer sought cosmetic surgery. I no longer tried to look like someone else. I came to accept myself.

Recently, a client, call her "Angela," came to me from the telesummit (she had bought my anti-aging program). We had a 30-minute session.

"How can I help you?"

We were on Skype, so I could see her; clearly, she had had plastic surgery to the point where she looked unreal: liposuction, breast implants, nose jobs…yet, she did not look good. She was in her early 60s, looking younger, but odd.

"We are going to connect with your higher self, to get to the truth. We will have to deal with what is true. OK?"

"I want that."

"You are not really overweight."

"I know, but I cannot bear to see myself in the mirror. I am taking Prozac. I'm depressed."

I understood she wanted to look like a Barbie doll, as I once wanted myself.

I made my sounds to re-direct her energy. "My sounds will help you make up your own mind about the wisdom of these surgeries."

"Wow! You know that I have over-done this."

"It's been a strain on you, going through these surgeries. Wouldn't you like a clearer mind?"

"Yes, I'd like that."

"You have other gifts to bring to the world, rather than just reshaped pictures of yourself."

Clearly, she had been obsessed with her looks. She claimed to be overweight, when she in fact looked fine. She was trying to overcome childhood influences. She told me about her childhood. Her mother was a constant dieter, always dressed to the nines. Angela saw her as perfect. Sadly, her mother did not reassure Angela about her own appearance.

"Shall we clear some of this?" I asked.

"Yes, I'd like to."

I made some of my vocalizations. "How do you feel now?"

"More peaceful. I have been worrying about what changes to make in my looks next."

"I'm clearing your unconscious mind. We are clearing out the ideas

     HAPPINESS MADE CRYSTAL CLEAR!

that you don't like about yourself. Think about all these negativities about your looks and your life."

After a few minutes, I told her to stop thinking about them. "Now, breathe deeply and release these ideas."

I could see her doing this, breathing deeply anyway.

"Angela, take a couple more deep breaths. How do you feel?"

"Wow! For the first time in my life, I feel at peace. My mind is actually calm. I had been thinking about my next surgery, and I don't have to do that anymore."

"Over the next few days, these thoughts will be removed from you. You will stop thinking about your weight and your looks. I am going to make some sounds. Release the energy you feel."

I made some more clearing sounds. When I finished, "How do you feel after this second clearing?"

"I feel that I am OK, and I am different. I feel empowered. I know I have had this pattern from my childhood, and I know I do not have to be perfect."

We did another clearing, to help her forgive her mother, who had been trying to help her, even though mistaken about what was best for her.

"I feel at peace for the first time in my life." She looked in the mirror. "Oh, my God, I look peaceful!"

"Let me know how things go for you. You will be open to new ideas and new options. Your true gifts will become clearer to you. If it feels good, follow it, as your Higher Power will help."

I have not heard from her; I hope she has been able to preserve the tranquility she had with me. Her body might not hold up to more operations.

She was putting herself in danger with this obsession. The shift in her attitude that occurred in our session has the possibility of saving her life.

Many clients come to me for physical problems that often end up being caused by something other than illness or injury. The breakthroughs help them realize there is more to life than worrying about its physical and material aspects. They learn they want to connect with their souls and their true selves. Once they do this, they have lives far better than before, and even their hearts and lungs respond to the change in their thinking. I often see this shift, and I am pleased when they say they are happier and healthier than ever before.

  HAPPINESS MADE CRYSTAL CLEAR!

Chapter 12

Talent

"A really great talent finds its happiness in execution."
– Johan Wolfgang Goethe

"True happiness involves the full use of one's power
and talents." *– John W. Gardner*

WHILE THERE IS pleasure in being a success due to a talent you possess, you may well find your greatest happiness during those periods when you are exercising your talent, rather than when you are being rewarded for it.

Doing well at what you are doing pleases you. You do not have to depend on the approval of others. There is a satisfaction in the action and a reward in the result, whether it leads to fame and fortune or not.

I have found that helping people with their pain or fear or anxiety or other problems has brought me more personal happiness than I ever could have predicted.

I worked with Jasmine recently, a woman in her late 50s. She was calling me from New York City. She obtained a program of mine, Unlimited Energy, from a telesummit. She liked the topic. This may have been the only telesummit she had ever heard…she was guided to me. We had a 30-minute phone session.

"Hi, Jasmine, this is Dawn. Thank you for trusting me to assist you. How can I help?"

"I'm married, with a couple of kids. I'm an orchestra musician, a violinist. I go all over the world to play. At 40, I married, to a man who is not a musician. I love him deeply. We have two children, now 8 and 10 years old. I am the primary breadwinner with my profession. Unfortunately, I feel a lot of pressure. I have high expenses. I'm tired. The tours wear me out. It was exciting when I was single, but now I'd like to be more of a mother and homemaker. I understand that I have to use this musical talent, but touring is getting wearing. I need a change. I am exhausted. I was drawn to your work, and I hope to be re-charged."

I started to study her energy. She was an empath, quite sensitive to the feelings of others. On her rare days off, sometimes she would unwind in the City by going to Central Park. "That's a wise choice. You've been doing so much traveling and feel so much pressure, you are getting worn down. Nature can help restore you."

"Yes. We are trying to live a good life in the City, but it is very expensive,

     HAPPINESS MADE CRYSTAL CLEAR!

and I want advanced schooling for the kids, plus a vacation. It is getting tiring."

"Do you and your husband really need to live this way? Have you discussed it? It sounds like you might do better to move out of the City, to somewhere less expensive, so you do not have to work quite so hard to cover your expenses."

"Yes. That make sense. Using my talent has worn me out. I think I need a change. I heard your program, and it appealed to me."

"Well, life is a journey, and sometimes we do have to change directions. I sense that your soul wants a change; it has had some damage from your childhood, where your parents pressured you to perform to your maximum"

"Agreed. I know they meant well, but now I find it hard to shut down. I am always looking for the next gig to help pay the bills."

"We are going to clear some of this childhood influence. Forgive your parents; they had your best interests at heart, but they were mistaken to pressure you. These old beliefs about achievement need to be cleared."

I did my sound therapy, moving her energy above her head, and I could sense that her own sounds themselves had changed.

"Jasmine, do you feel something changing?"

"Yes, a weight is lifting from my shoulders, and I find I am breathing more fully. I feel less high-strung."

We did some more energy movement.

"And what about now?"

"I feel something has shifted, that I have been a robot, enjoying nothing. When I am with my family, I am worrying about making money with my music. I feel so much better!"

I showed her how to create an energy boundary around herself, a bubble of light to protect herself, to make others have less influence on her.

"Jasmine, this boundary will help you feel more peaceful and make your mind feel clearer. You might want to spend less time with the orchestra and more time with your family and nature."

We did some additional energy clearing and grounding to planet Earth, and I could tell she was doing better.

"I've just grounded your energy," I told her.

"Oh! My mind is not racing any more. I am breathing more deeply. It feels miraculous. It's no wonder that I found you. It seems a miracle that I listened to the telesummit. I will listen to another telesummit with you soon.'"

I am looking forward to hearing from Jasmine. I am confident she is going to have a happier time now that she has been cleared of some of these harmful energy influences.

Chapter 13

LOVE

"Mink Schmink, Money Schmoney,
Think you're hot now, don't ya honey?
What have you got if you haven't got love?

….Happiness is not a thing you can buy.
It takes loving, lotsa loving, from the right guy."
Eartha Kitt, song "Mink Schmink" by *Sidney Cutner and Leo Shuken*

"I was lookin' for love in all the wrong places
Lookin' for love in too many faces…."
Johnny Lee, song *Looking for Love* by *Bob Morrison, Wanda Mollette, and Pam Ryan*

I myself have been "looking for love in all the wrong places." I had my first boyfriend at age 14. He was 16. I never had a parent, advisor, or mentor to tell me to wait until I became older. Lee was a Southern boy, very popular, a drummer in a rock and roll band whom I met in school. It was the 1980s and rock-and-roll, "big-hair bands," were popular. I had my hair lacquered up high. I thought this was love. We dated all through high school, and it ended when I was 20, dating about seven years, leading to a pregnancy and an abortion. In fact, the relationship was empty. I was so insecure. Looks were key, and I worried about not measuring up .

Next was a man I met at my job. Randy was a V.P. at the plastics company, much more than 10 years older than I. A father figure? He enjoyed having a younger woman on his arm, "arm candy," and he bought me expensive gifts, including a motorcycle. That affair lasted 8 years. I found him too obsessive and controlling, and I had trouble getting out of the relationship. Warning: don't date your boss! I broke up with him as I quit the company.

Then I started working at the police department. I dated my partner. Steve and I spent over eight hours a day in the car together. He broke up with his steady girl. We married. Not controlling, approximately my age, not a father figure, but someone safe. His subsequent blinding eye injury wrecked our marriage. He could no longer work at the police department, and he became very angry, trying to get a big settlement, ending up with a small one. His anger undermined our relationship. When the money came it, we split it…and we split.

Next came "Sam," a customer at my tanning salon business. I was still getting over Steve. Sam and I married ,and he quickly became dependent on me, a total disaster, an alcoholic, a real psychopath, having hidden his true personality. His boozing cost him his job. Soon, he stayed away from home overnights. He became disabled

   HAPPINESS MADE CRYSTAL CLEAR!

through a motorcycle accident. I had it! I knew that these relationships were doing me no good. I gave Sam almost everything, and I left for Hawaii.

The moral is: I did not experience unconditional love from my family, nor from my romantic interests. I've been looking for love in the wrong places. I should have looked to myself, known myself.

Even when homeless, I found I could be happy without having someone to love me. I can find my own happiness inside me. I can love myself, my own soul, my own heart. This turned my life around. It healed me.

I've been happily single for 15 years, and I find love with my pets and from myself, from my inside-out. If I meet another man I find interesting, I will know when it is the real thing. I don't want the empty relationships I used to have. Any future relationship will have to be as equals, as people who are not needy but who can support themselves and aid each other.

This week I had a client, Diane. She got one of my programs. Her session focused on her marriage. She is seeking a divorce from a husband who has been putting her down over their eight years of marriage. He even cheated on her. Fortunately, they no longer live together.

She needed my help clearing the negative energy she had gotten from his jealousy and criticism. She felt stuck. She needs him to pay her child support. To complicate things, he lost his job due to cheating with a coworker. Sadly, she still loves him, and she has had trouble moving forward.

Much of this dependency started with the absence of a father figure while she was growing up. This made her clingy. Her parents passed her on to others for her care as a child. Unsurprisingly, her neediness contributed to breaking up the marriage.

I advised her to move from her too-expensive apartment to something more affordable. With that change, her money problems would diminish. She needs a better job. Her education was excellent, in a financial field, and she could get a better position, now that she would not be co-dependent on her husband.

She needs to get child support for the two children. She felt she was sinking in quicksand, and I helped remove fearful emotions. We disposed of some of the toxic energy…clearing it, clearing her conscious mind. She felt better. She came to several positive conclusions during our session: she will change her job, change her location, get the child support, and wrap up the divorce. She realized she did not have to be so dependent on her husband.

She said she felt much calmer when we were done. She thanked me for the session. She had started off crying a lot, and this tapered off. She knows she will now be fine by herself. She is going to call me in a month and tell me how it works out.

I find that many of my clients are in relationships not good for them. Often, they stay for financial reasons. They also often have insecurity underlying their personality. They have a lot to offer, but they don't realize that. We clear out the traumas and insecurities to find their true gifts, so they can get out of situations that are holding them down and let them find their own true happiness from within. Sometimes, they will find a truly beneficial love once the toxic one

    HAPPINESS MADE CRYSTAL CLEAR!

has been abandoned. They will have made room for another person in their life.

Confidence increases when negative energies are removed, and my clients find that they can do much more than they once thought they could.

Chapter 14

LUCK

"Luck is a matter of preparation meeting opportunity." – *Lucius Annaeus Seneca*

"Luck? I don't know anything about luck. I've never banked on it, and I'm afraid of people who do. Luck to me is something else: Hard work - and realizing what is opportunity and what isn't." – *Lucille Ball*

"When I've least expected it, an enormous opportunity or stroke of luck has crossed right under my nose. So, I tell everybody, if you're passionate about what you do, and you love it, do it. But do your homework. Because you'll never know when the opportunity is going to happen." – *Julie Andrews*

[All three "luck" quotes were obtained from https://www.brainyquote. com.]

BEING ABLE TO read this book means you have already had unusual good luck. You have been born in this century or the previous one, have the physical skills to be able to read, and the education to understand it. You have likely been born in a civilized, advanced country, and even if you are only middle-class in income, you are among the world's wealthiest. You are the outcome of the DNA lottery, where you could have been a sibling rather than yourself. So, consider yourself lucky!

Will luck bring happiness? Sad to say, many who are lucky as described above view themselves as insufficiently lucky, compared to others, or even as unlucky, because of bad breaks that have befallen them: an accident, a disability, a divorce, firing, disappointment…. We can always find others who seem luckier than we are, and that line of thought will only bring unhappiness.

Instead, recognize that some outcomes depend mostly on our own doing, and some clearly do not. We do the best we can, "play the cards we are dealt" as well as we can, enjoy what we can, and accept that we will win some and lose some due to luck. We can improve our odds by heeding the wisdom of those who say that good luck attends those of us who meet opportunity with prior preparation, "doing our homework."

Most of my life I saw myself as a victim. Why was I born here? In this chaos? I seemed unlucky, but I dreamed of winning the lottery. Money was the goal, as my mom raised six kids on welfare. From age 9 with my first job to my later years, I sought money to make our family happy. Money, money, money! It was supposed to be the key. My paper route was gotten to help myself and the family. I felt bad for my mom, who wanted better things for us.

I was a hard worker, trying to make as much money as possible. In school, however, I was tired from working after school. I had no mentors. I came to class after uproar at home.

In my twenties, my police job was a blessing, though not a big money-maker. Even though I did have more money, there was no ”aha!” moment, no being happy simply due to the money I made.

I was even more financially successful during my second marriage and two businesses, but the marriage itself was dysfunctional, and I hit rock-bottom. Clearly, money was not my key to happiness.

After the divorce and having shed my possessions, becoming a homeless person, I found I was no happier than before, even though I once had more money. Money luck, good or bad, was not the key.

In Hawaii, even though homeless, I finally found myself happy. I connected with my Higher Self, true happiness.

Now, after twenty-five years, I am in a better situation, and I am known internationally, fortunately with enough money, yet this is not what has made me happy. Other things count more. I could lose my money and still be happy.

Luck? How does this connect with luck? I realized that being lucky, which meant having money to me, did not guarantee happiness.

Luck is being alive, being able to walk this Earth, breathe easily, enjoying my health. This brings me happiness.

A recent client, Jamie, was a Skype caller who got an anti-aging program.

"I just want to look younger!" She exclaimed right at the start.

"Anything going on with you, Jamie?"

"I want to be luckier in life. I've got my mom's genes, her cellulite around my thighs, her sagging chin, and her flabby neck." She connected luck with looking good rather than with having money. Certainly, genes are luck and genes greatly influence our attractiveness.

"How old are you?"

"I'm 62, married for decades, but I feel I am losing myself, getting less attractive."

"Jamie, do you feel you are not lucky?"

"Yes, my friends are all better looking. Skinny! My husband is demanding. He's rich and I've been 'arm candy,' and I don't want to lose him to a better-looking woman."

"Let's discuss why you feel unlucky."

She was obviously obsessed with her looks, and we needed to work on this. After all, I had once been that way myself, even trying risky surgery to improve my appearance.

"Jamie, we are all going to age. I see you on the Skype picture, and you look quite good. You are thinking you are unlucky, but this is not necessarily true."

"I do need to drop my belief system. I am too busy working on my looks. I am tired, and maybe I am not paying as much attention to my husband as I should."

"Yes, you are creating your own unhappiness. You are lucky to be alive and healthy. You must value this."

She stated to cry, as she had been paying so much attention to her looks and not thinking about things of more substance. She was chasing youth, and this can be dangerous. For example, her stem cell surgery was not successful.

"I cannot keep searching for the next procedure to transform my looks."

"Right. These operations can be dangerous, and you may be unlucky with the outcome. All these beliefs about looks --- that you must be pretty to be happy --- are wrong."

We spent some extra time on these beliefs to help her rid herself of them.

"Keep a journal, focus on what you want. Put your energy into your true talents and how to help other people."

We had a final grounding session, and I could tell she was much less anxious and nervous at the end.

"I feel like a new person. Relaxed. I don't have to change myself to be happy."

"This clearing will continue for the next few days."

She thanked me for the call.

In our situations, we have ideas about what was luck, and these beliefs are often mistaken, as luck is not money or good looks, because we can be happy without money and without being pretty. Luck is coming into personal power and being better connected with the Higher Power and with our souls.

Peace, health, and happiness…luck!

Chapter 15

PETS

"Animals are such agreeable friends – they ask no questions, they pass no criticisms." – *George Eliot*

"Such short little lives our pets have to spend with us, and they spend most of it waiting for us to come home each day." – *John Grogan*

"Until one has loved an animal, a part of one's soul remains unawakened." – *Anatole France*

These quotations (from www.dodo.com) highlight how much our pets give us, how important we are to them, and how little they ask for in return. Our animal companions can be true blessings.

As I mentioned, in my early life I had been mostly by myself, almost without friends, an outcast. I lived in a lower-middle-class neighborhood, and my family was looked down upon. My one friend had a mother who was a screamer. That did not last long.

Fluffy, a hamster, was my first pet, my best friend. He lived four years. My mother would not let me have a dog; she said the food was "too expensive." We were on welfare, so she had a point. I could be myself with the wild animals I met outside, like a female Dr. Dolittle, who "talked to the animals." They were not judgmental. When I brought animals in from the outside, my mother would throw them out. "Food doesn't grow on trees over here," she'd scream.

On my own, years later, I always had a dog. My dogs accepted me. I accepted them. Unconditionally. Yes, pets are not the ultimate happiness, but they are a positive element, a complement to our living here on Earth. We learn from them that happiness can come from simple things; our pets appreciate food and shelter and some petting…content, without talking back.

A client, "Mildred," bought a healing package of mine recently, "Get out of Pain Forever." She bought it primarily for herself, but at the scheduling of the session, she asked if I could heal one of her pets, too. I agreed.

"Hi, Dawn, I bought your program, but I have an older dog, thirteen years old, with a hip issue. We have been using natural remedies, and I thought maybe you could help my dog with his pain. You mentioned you work with animals."

"Sure, let's get started with you, and we'll work with your dog at the end."

"I've been married 28 years; we live in a rural area, with eight cats, seven dogs, and eight parrots. They keep me busy! My husband and I don't talk much. These pets bring me happiness. I really want to help this sick dog. His hip is bothering him."

First, I had a regular session with Mildred. "Your pets are great, but it sounds to me like they are causing you to work too hard. This takes time away from yourself and from your family. Do you have some talents, some gifts you want to pursue?"

"Not really. I want to spend my efforts on my pets."

"I sense that you need some better balance to your life. You have taken on the caretaker role, for pets and for relatives, and you have forgotten to care for yourself."

"True, I grew up in an unhappy family, and I did not enjoy myself except when I was working with pets. Now, I'd like to have a more peaceful and happier, more satisfying and fulfilling life."

"You have put a barrier on your feelings. They are stopped up in your stomach area, and you are not in touch with your own true feelings. We can address that."

"Yes, I'd like to feel freer and make choices that bring me more happiness."

"Your son and husband should pitch in to help you more. You'll have to set some boundaries, especially with your son, whom you describe as not helping out. Give him some chores, some responsibility."

"I agree. Hearing it from you convinces me I have to change this part of my life."

     HAPPINESS MADE CRYSTAL CLEAR!

We cleared her unconscious mind, using my sounds. She had been afraid to be herself. "You have to find yourself. I am giving you some added energy to use to take action with."

"I'm ready, and I'm glad I found you." She was ready for me to work with her ailing pooch.

She brought her dog close to the telephone. Skippy, a big Labrador Retriever, had sympathetically taken on some of Mildred's emotions, trying to comfort her.

When I told Mildred this, she replied, "I knew that Skippy was special."

I could tell his energy was blocked in his back legs. I did some sound therapy. When he rose after the session, he walked much better, according to Mildred, who was pleased.

We did a bit more work to end her session. For herself, she planned to get out more and to try some new things.

Later, she wrote me that her life was changing for the good, and that Skippy was doing better. Her son agreed he should be contributing more to the household. The energy of the home was being redistributed positively.

I truly believe that pets are a great addition to our lives. They bring depth, bring us closer to Nature, help us simplify our lives, showing us how basic life can be. Having pets is a plus, but we must care for ourselves first, which is where our happiness comes form. The outside factors in our lives, like pets, complement our inner lives, to form a complete whole, bringing everything together…and in balance.

Chapter 16

GRATITUDE

"He is a wise man who does not grieve for the things which he has not, but rejoices for those which he has."
— *Epictetus*

"Reflect upon your present blessings, of which every man has plenty; not on your past misfortunes, of which all men have some." — *Charles Dickens*

"You say grace before meals. All right. But I say grace before the concert and the opera, and grace before the play and pantomime, and grace before I open a book, and grace before sketching, painting, swimming, fencing, boxing, walking, playing, dancing and grace before I dip the pen in the ink." — *G. K. Chesterton*

"There are only two ways to live your life. One is as

though nothing is a miracle. The other is as though everything is a miracle." — *Albert Einstein*

[from https://daringtolivefully.com/gratitude-quotes]

WHEN I WAKE up each day in lovely Maui, I think of all the blessings I have been given, and I am thankful.

Almost all of us have much to be thankful for, and a thankful heart is a happy heart. Gratitude makes today better and tomorrow better still. So, "count your blessings," and your life will be even happier.

I feel that in my life, even to early adulthood, I was pretty much a victim, blamng others for my struggle, the lack of love, my looks I dis-liked. I was angry and unhappy. I was depressed, which I tried to fight with anti-depressants, which messed my body up. My emotions were trapped. I became numb. Then my gift came to me, and I became a healer, first healing myself, then helping others.

I was working at various jobs, while learning more about myself and healing myself. The guidance I got seems to have come from my Creator, and it accelerated my personal healing. Helping others helped me. The universe does pay one back.

This went on for many years. I became alive, no longer emotionally shut down. Now, I can feel more deeply. As I matured, I see my life has been a path of progress with a reason, and I am not a victim but a victor, and I now help others to become victorious.

Moving from my dark place into the light, I have learned gratitude for the simplest things in life: my breath, my heartbeat, my health, just being alive, and finding my true self. It was hard, and I would not choose to repeat all this, but it has been worth doing to get to where I am now. I waken every day with a thank-you to my Creator!

With my clients, I try to help them see, beyond the veil of illusion, the truth of the basic happiness available to them. We work together to manifest our blessings: "I do have a lucky life. I could otherwise be a person starving in Africa!"

Gratitude is a higher state of energetic vibration, and sharing it with others brightens the world in your vicinity. People who meet you pick up on this, and their moods are elevated by yours. As we rise, so does our world.

     HAPPINESS MADE CRYSTAL CLEAR!

Jack Canfield Interviews *Pain Free* Author Dawn Crystal

Douglas Winslow Cooper, Ph.D.

An alternative to medical treatment for pain was discussed with Dawn Crystal by Jack Canfield, author of the *New York Times* multi-million-selling book series *Chicken Soup for the Soul.*

Before the interview, Dawn Crystal applied her voice-sound treatment techniques to a painful neck and back condition Canfield was suffering.

"You did something…healing my neck," he comments on the recording of their session, https://video.wixstatic.com/video/14f4a3_1e0aff9 01cf24ec0806d437c4a4f5b91/1080p/mp4/file.mp4.

"Yes. Voice-sound healing is something I do with my voice….I found my gift at the lowest point of my life….Sounds that came from my heart."

Canfield asked for examples of her successes. A lady she treated at the woman's bedside had been turning blue. After going to the hospital, she returned and thanked Dawn for saving her life.

Dawn believes her sounds move energy through the body. Chinese call it "chi" or "qi," an internal energy that needs to be unblocked. One of her specialties is anti-aging. Her mp3 recordings can help her listeners.

You can get more information about her techniques at DawnCrystalHealing.com, where this interview is also.

Canfield ended the interview this way, "I am someone who believes in this kind of thing…I am somewhat skeptical, and I was pretty impressed.…Most people are suffering from some kind of pain…they should check it out."

Testimonials

Dear Dawn,

Many thanks for the session. It was very helpful and powerfully healing. My back is a lot better as though I had a break in the middle of my body (legs and trunk) and it has gone back as one piece and what you told me about moving forward and my husband made a lot of sense. And especially healing the lack of consciousness. I do feel more connected and centered and really trust that I can move forward.

M

Hi Dawn,

I am thrilled to have a private session with you again. My life completely changed as a result of our work together. With immense gratitude,

A

Thank You so much, I am so grateful for this mp3 of sound healing. It soothed and relaxed me. I am truly grateful for the kindness and love you share!

Namaste
G

Hi

I love your work & really feel & see the benefits of doing the liposuction mp3 .... it's totally out there, weird & wacky, it's amazing! Far better than going for surgery, fillers etc!

I live in the UK & we really don't get much sun. As part of your beauty & rejuv packages, I wondered if you could do an mp3 for a sun tan without having to go to the tanning salon or holiday in the sun .... it sounds crazy but if anyone could do it you could. Hope you can help, this would be a huge success considering the size of the tanning/fake tan industry.

With Blessings,
M

Amazon 5-star review of *FEAR FREE:*

Dawn Crystal is an amazing Sound Healer! This is her second book and it is just as wonderful as the first! I have also had the good fortune to experience personal healings from Dawn through the Learning Strategies Corporation "Silent Clearings" program for 2 years in a row. Her next "Silent Clearings" program is expected to start around February 19 or so. In addition, she also has a wonderful website and I have purchased a number of her programs from there as well. I cannot wait for Dawn to come out with her "Complete Dental Health" energy healing program on her website. Through Dawn, I have been healed of lifelong anxiety and panic-attacks (I am 50), as well as a painful back and right shoulder that have been bothering me for many years! She is truly amazing and a really wonderful person as well. I feel very lucky to have found her and I look forward to many years of Dawn's healing programs in my life. Thank you for everything, Dawn! You are a life-saver and you deserve every happiness! Much love to you always. You have a True Gift and I feel so lucky to have experienced your healing directly. Aloha! :-)

L

This work has been so potent that the quality of my voice has elevated and I am now a produced composer and singer.

My relationships are healed and I have overcome patterns that I thought would take years to work through.

The emotional releasing was intense , more so on the 2nd or 3rd day of clearing.

I did the whole upgrade and harmful environments , as well as liposuction.

My body is free from cellulite and varicose veins (which was absolutely not the case before this) and my skin looks and feels better than ever.

I am living a completely new life, feeling like a lighter magical being constantly surrounded by miracles.

D

Hi Dawn,

This is a testimonial for the 30-minute session we had. I was amazed at how quickly you honed into the core issues bothering me. Even though it wasn't easy to hear, I knew in my heart that you spoke the truth. Clearing the emotional issues you identified will no doubt heal my physical problems faster.

Thank you Dawn!
K

Hello, I have purchased Dawn's Weight Loss and Anti-Aging Programs, as well as have had a session with Dawn. In the session Dawn was able to locate the blocked energy in my body without me telling her where the pain was. I could feel the energy move out through my body, giving me more energy and feeling lighter. Through the years I have tried many healing modalities; none of them have worked as quickly as Dawn's has. Looking forward to another session with Dawn.

R

Dawn,

I purchased four of your products, but I got a session with only one of them (would have rocked to buy sessions with all of them). I had been using the products before my session, and they did help. However, the session with you, really blew me away. I have never felt light like that before in my whole life. Totally awesome. The information that you gave me during the session was also really beneficial and I can see immediate results with use. Everything you said was right from my higher self and I know it. That gave me a lot of direction and new-found sense of self. I feel more in tune with myself than I ever have and it's only going to get better. If this is what happens in one session, I cannot imagine what would happen in more.

B

Hi Dawn,

I would like to share with my experience in using your anti-aging program

the mp3s are amazingly powerful , I felt the change instantly after each time I listen to them and after a time of using them every few weeks I have a glowing skin and healthy hair, plus that I feel emotionally and physically stronger and have more energy through the day.

Thank you so much for your amazing healing.

Love you,
R

Hi Dawn: I bought Total Body Rejuvenation package. I was shocked by the immediate results I saw the very first time when I listened to Healthy Hair, Skin & Nails. My skin was glowing and the nails looks like I had gotten it done professionally. My knees are doing much better also.

Thank you very much for the personal session. You were so kind, and resolved lots of personal family issues coming from generation.

Love,
C

Hi Dawn,

I have not purchased any of your products yet. I do have some recordings from your old webinars. I especially love the energy clearing work that you do in the webinar and listen to it daily. I feel at a level of higher vibration after listening to it.

Thank you for sharing.
S

Dear Dawn,

I have bought some of your packages and I can say that your work is awesome! The recordings have helped me feel so much better. I have some serious issues with my back, but after hearing your recordings the pain has subsided, so I know it's working! You are a blessing and thank you for sharing your gift to help the world. I can't wait to experience my private session with you!

With much love,
P

     HAPPINESS MADE CRYSTAL CLEAR!

Hi Dawn,

I just wanted to say that you are so insightful and gifted. You knew so much of my 'story' and quickly intuited who was draining my energy, where I was losing it, and how to stop it. You were able to see where I held stress in my body and released it for me. I say prayers of gratitude every morning, and I now include having known you along my journey as part of that. Thank you for your heart-felt intentions, and the clearings I received. I listen to your MP3's almost daily now, and can see how I am looking and feeling younger every day. I have truly been telling so many about you and your gift of sound healings. You are an inspiration. From one light worker to another....thank you dear Soul for sharing your gift with us so beautifully.

I.

Hello,

I purchased Dawn's Anti Aging program the end of the year; previously I purchased the Weight Loss program.

Have gone through all the package items for the Weight Loss and just a couple of the Anti Aging. Wanted to say that I feel that I have more energy; old energy is clearing out which is awesome!!!

I had a session with Dawn in December from the purchase of Weight Loss. I need to schedule another one I purchased with the Anti Aging program. After my December 3rd session, I had emailed asking about pets. Was told if ever book another session could share some of it with my animals....

Thank you for your time.

Blessings,
R

Hi dawn my name is C*******, Thank you so so much for taking the time to do this awesome call I am so happy and so grateful that you did record this because in the email I received it didn't have a time and didn't know when to tune in for it, I have listened to the replay and the energy was amazing!! Looking forward to the one-day retreat in February with Erma FHTJ, I will be there virtually, although live would be awesome I am sure it will be just as awesome to be able to listen in to you and all the others for a full day of clearings, activations and amazing knowledge and tools. Thanks again Big Hugs Love and Blessings

C

I worked with Dawn to help me increase my energy. I have always had an issue with an energy dip during the mid-afternoon. Dawn helped me clear what was holding my life force energy down. Since my session with Dawn, I am amazed! I have had a steady amount of energy every single day since the session. I don't need short afternoon naps anymore!!! For my work - this is awesome! I am much more productive during the day so I am able to end my workday earlier. Everyone in my family is so much happier because of this! Thank you Dawn!!!

Dear Dawn,

Happy New Year!

I have a big testimonial for you, after purchasing total body rejuvenation and anti-aging. I listen faithfully to them, and at night for your best sleep item! Now though, my computer has crashed and I cannot find them ! Please help, only when they are not there do I realize how reliant I have been, in their helping me keep in shape in body and

 HAPPINESS MADE CRYSTAL CLEAR!

mind. No one can guess my age and I feel great, but please advise if they can be resent as I do not want to be without them for long!

I purchased through Eram Saed and Judy I think!

Love and light,
S

~~

Dear Dawn,

I am so happy to get your 2 packages: No more pain and Anti-aging. I was so hungry to listen and experience your all mp3.

I can say that all the pain of feeling and emotions and heart-broken pain just disappeared in a miraculous way. I feel so good now and I'm expecting more good things to happen… I'm able to wear a dress which I was unable to close the zip, my cravings almost gone… I look radiant and full of energy and I feel my face it is glowing and I'm happy to receive so many compliments in the office...or from people who know me.

I listen to the Clearing feeling and emotions mp3 for 5 days in row maybe 5 times a day and from the first day I felt improvement….it soothe my heart …. So happy for that…

I listen to your life story and your sincerity of your story and it has just amazed me the way you went through all your life… I am so inspired by you.

Thank you, Patty, Carry, and

Thank you, Dawn, for being part of my life.

Best Regards,
A

Sharjah, UAE

This is my 2nd session with you!! The session we had last night was incredible. I had to lay down for 2 hours. My head and body felt a buzzing sensation. It was also trance like. The work we did letting go of the abuse with my father was freeing in a way I never experienced before. I feel more love for him! I didn't realize how much I needed to hear that he was sorry for his part in our relationship. As for my husband, I'm seeing things differently!! I want to take back my power more than ever!! Dawn, thank you dearly for your love, support and healing!!! You told me a few times that I am an old soul with a beautiful spirit!! You said not to let it go to my ego, and it hasn't. My heart and spirit needed to know and hear that my light is bright!! It isn't something that I feel that I'm better than anyone!! I never felt better than anyone, in fact just the opposite!! I look forward to strengthening my boundaries in our next session! I need more confidence in myself in all areas. But especially "making it on my own". I still feel like a little weak girl in that area! I know that God has put you in my path; I am immensely grateful to him for that! Thank you again!! Can't wait for our next session!! I'm sending you a whole bunch of love to your beautiful spirt!! Big hugs too!!

J

Hi Dawn,

Here's my testimonial for wonderful experiences with your healing voice.

Please edit or re-write to suit your needs.

First, I purchased the Anti-aging Package. Then purchased Facial, followed by Pain Free.

I had chronic fatigue for many years. Have released, detoxed, healed with other healers and master's for many years but kept coming back. With one amazing healer, my fatigue was getting better but mild attacks came back. That's when I met your healing voice.

With the Anti-aging program my inflammation went away after listening for a few days and became more energetic to live with vitality every day.

For those that may have similar symptoms this really means a great deal.

My boyfriend had pain in his hand from joint pain/inflammation. He purchased the Pain Free program and now no more pain and the inflammation is gone. Every time the weather pattern changed, he was suffering. This was a symptom which was hereditary (came from lineage). So, It's magic.

I also had a private session which I highly recommend for everybody as Dawn really sees the whole you, sees the deep core emotional issues and releases it heals immediately.

The Pain program, while it is specific to the pain of different parts of the body it is recommended for any symptom without physical pain.

The healing addresses whatever you may need both physically and emotionally at the time you listen.

I have been listening to these healings for a few months and my body tingles more profoundly today. I feel lighter.

An amazing healing method beyond Sound/voice, enabling you to reach the Source yourself.

PS Pain Free - when you say pain free one usually thinks of physical pains. You should stress that your healing really focuses into emotional pains as well. I saw "scenes" leaving.

Another thing. Regarding your book, I have an account with Amazon Japan and without purchasing from them I cannot write a comment. So I'm asking how this can be done.

I am soooooo grateful and thankful to have met you Dawn. Please create MP3s for "eyes" and Immunity for all seasons and cold/flu in the winter season.

Mahalo with love,
H

The first time I experienced Dawn Crystal, I was sitting on a chair resting my chronically painful knees. I was tired and dosed off, but was suddenly awoken by one of her loud, high pitched vocalizations.

I began to laugh...NOT at Dawn (I did not question her sincerity), but because I was so startled! After listening to the rest of Dawn's interview and receiving her remote Energy Healing offerings, I got up from my chair, and noticed that my Knees did **NOT** hurt!

Did Dawn's Sound Healing help my knees, I wondered ?!? I ordered Dawn's "Total Body Rejuvenation" program to experiment and find out.

After listening to Dawn's Recordings, my Knees felt stronger, more stable, and **Pain FREE!** WOW!!

A couple of weeks later, I experienced another (not the first time) bout with Vertigo, Nausea and lack of Balance. I had a phone session with

Dawn during this time, and she saw and cleared blockages in my upper Chakras, and Grounded me very deeply so I felt much more Balanced and stable when I walked.

Dawn also saw causes of some of my physical and emotional issues going back to my Family and lineage, and she helped clear them. I would wholeheartedly recommend Dawn Crystal for her miraculous Healing programs and personal sessions.

Besides Dawn's amazing Healing Gifts, she has great integrity and compassion, and humbly gives credit to GOD for any healing that others receive through her work.

MANY THANKS & MANY BLESSINGS to you, Dawn.
- N

The words seem empty to describe the profound impact of my session with Dawn. She has an amazing ability to listen to the soul speak and is guided by Pure Source. In my short 25 or 30 minutes with her I was able to heal 30 year old emotional wounds I didn't even realize were still there! The impact on my life has been a delightful effervescent emotional resilience that I was unaware I wasn't enjoying !!

Strongly recommend you enjoy any opportunity to do individual work with her, no matter what you may intend, she has a direct link to pure source that will allow you to have your intention attended to - yet not limited by your vision of what you need. An incredible experience to be able to have Source work directly with you, through her pervasive nurturing healing gift!!

- M

Weight loss program: Using the Mp3s brought much awareness to parts of my body and perceptions I had that were not what I wanted. These help to clear and reprogram old patterns. My 1 on 1 session was phenomenal. I felt much lighter as I let go of many attachments/chords!

MK

Aloha Dawn Crystal,

You are so amazing! I just happened to catch you on Quantum Conversations today and as I was listening you gave me a personal reading, like you and I separated from the show and had a cup of tea together, you are really to the point and down to business, made me cry, and I just look at you and see Hawaiian Royalty, an Ascended Master, and Lemurian Honcho! (and mermaid!) Plus, you are so beautiful and brilliant.

Wow, what a gift to get a glimpse of who you are, your photo is very powerful, and a healing tool! I wish I could remember everything you said to me, you gave me the gift of taking off a blindfold, you said I was wearing a blindfold and couldn't see who I really am.

I look forward to the unfolding. At the moment I am a poet, and here is a poem about you!

Dawn Crystal
ever insightful
full of grace
with a flower in her hair
she rises above the ocean waves
she resides in the mountain
presides over the whales, dolphins
mystic reveler
bubbles at her feet
she is alive
freedom between her sounds
the ocean vibrates with her
momentum she is garnished
by the leis threaded by all of her children
she has healed
for she is the great one
that all man has known for many ages
she smiles because she knows
she knows.
Love you, F. D.

Hello Dawn - I purchased your Weight Loss Package. I have been listening for several days (not yet a week) and I lost 5 pounds without trying. Also my right knee pain has decreased and I feel I have more energy. I also have realized a positive shift in my self-image.

Thanks,

- J

Hello Crystal,

i have very hard water at the place where i live not so nice to drink.

when i use you energizing water mp3 on it, it becomes much softer and more alive.

J., Austria

It has only been a few days and just hit and miss listening to the modules and I lost 4 pounds and 1" off my waist so I look forward to the results as I continue to listen to them more regularly. I am grateful to have Sound Therapy available to assist with weight loss!

Thanks
S. E.

P.S. I look forward to more changes after I have my private session too!

I had heard Dawn several times on telesummits and, each time, I felt a strong resistance. Fortunately, I have figured out by now that resistance means there is something important for me there. Oh boy was I right!

My session with Dawn really blew me away. Everything she said was spot on and everything she did hit the mark; so much shifted in these 30 minutes! The positive impact of the shift was felt immediately on all levels – physical, emotional, spiritual, and it translated into a stream of "good news" coming through in the following days. In other words, there was a noticeable turnaround in my life as a whole after that session.

Although I bought the session as part of a weight loss package, its scope and impact were much broader. Dawn makes every minute of the 30-minute session count, without ever losing connection, warmth and compassion.

In terms of the weight loss package, I am still going through the MP3s, so it is early days. What I notice first and foremost at this time is a shift in approaching the issue and food choices specifically. I am quite confident that overall, the session and MP3s will translate into some positive results regarding weight.

I highly recommend Dawn Crystal. She is truly phenomenal.

V. M.

Hi Dawn,

I am in such deep gratitude to you and your amazing work.

I contacted you to work with my beloved dog and not only did he receive healing, I also got an amazing session with you.

You are a truly divine being and for anyone that is looking for healing... Dawn is an incredible healer...

Lots of love and gratitude
N

Dear Dawn,

I purchased all your energy downloads and have been playing them regularly since summer and I must say, they make me feel at peace and full of optimism. We also had two one on one session which I enjoyed immensely. My life has become more of experiencing trust and lightness which I am so very grateful for. You certainly have helped lifting much burden from my shoulders. Thank you so very much for your immense support!

May the light guide you at all times, always, much love
C

Part of me felt kind of stupid and crazy for signing up for this even though I've been using your programs for decades. I mean, I can't exactly afford it, and it's just some lady making weird noises over the phone. But my intuition kept urging me, so I went for it.

I'm almost 50 but had such an excruciating childhood, I've still suffered the effects no matter how hard I've tried everything under the sun to heal. Some things have helped but not enough to quell the constant underlying desire to end it. I thought about killing myself all the time as a kid, and the desire always remained no matter how hard I tried to heal and think positive. I would never do it because I wouldn't leave my child alone in the world, and I knew it was just leftover darkness, but to varying degrees it was the backdrop to even the happiest of times for my entire life.

Well, yesterday was Suicide prevention day, and I realized that I had not thought about killing myself for several days. That weight is gone. There's light in that place. So, that's pretty cool for only one session. Thanks for that. I'm excited to see what happens next.

L

                              HAPPINESS MADE CRYSTAL CLEAR!

Dear Dawn,

Being an energy healer, medical intuitive, empath, animal communicator myself, I can truly say that you are very gifted and that your sound healing frequencies are very strong and effective.

I thoroughly enjoyed the private session you so generously included in the purchase of your total body Rejuvenation program. It made me feel so much better, more grounded and alive. But most important I could feel your passion for your work. You truly want to be of service and your heart connection with the client is very strong. It has been an honor connecting with you via Skype.

Thank you, you are an inspiration for me.

With Angel blessings,
A

August was a particularly difficult month for me. Fortunately, I had my private session with Dawn on September 3rd. That session was phenomenal. I released much negative energy I didn't even know I had. That night, I had the first good night's sleep I have had in a long time. The dreams were positive, too, instead of ones about some tragedy or another that I had to overcome. I am currently working my way through the series of Abundance Blocks mp3's that were part of the package I bought and find them helpful as well. My energy is now more positive, and I wake up looking forward to how the day will unfold instead of thinking this is just another day I have to get through. Dawn is truly amazing. I connected with her energy during the webinar she was on and the connection became more evident when I spoke to her on the phone. You will not regret purchasing any of the packages she offers as she is sincere in wanting to help you and not just wanting to make a buck pushing a product you really don't need. She helps you find the true you that is part of the Whole/God. Once you find that part of you and learn how to allow what your desires to manifest instead of resisting those things you are attracting that you don't want, you will find your life has changed forever in a very, very positive way. I am truly grateful I found the one person who could get through my resistance and help me birth the part of me that is truly part of Source/God. Now I can continue exploring what is mine to do in this lifetime allowing only those energies that are in my highest good to manifest themselves in Divine timing. Dawn helped me, and she can help you, too, if you choose to allow that to happen.

D

I was in extreme pain back in the latter part of June/July. I do not know where it came from and why, and my appointment with Dawn was scheduled for July 21. I asked Dawn if she could move me up or squeeze me in because I was experiencing excruciating pain that I had never felt before. Since someone had rescheduled, she had an opening for the July 7, and I was able to take that spot. Dawn did what she does best with her sound healings and going to the core of the problem, I didn't even notice, but my pain went away and that next week, the pain was gone. It went as mysteriously as it came. It was miraculous. Thank you, Dawn, so much for your generosity and flexibility.

J

 HAPPINESS MADE CRYSTAL CLEAR!

Dawn,

You're a magical gift to my life. Finding you randomly one evening after being guided in a dream by my grandfather who I channel with often, he gave me a perfect description of the person who I needed for my next healing. That very next day in my inbox I received an email that had a replay of one of your online talks, I knew immediately seeing your picture you where the exact person my grandfather had described the night before so I proceeded to listen to your free healing followed by purchasing the get out of pain package which included a private session with you. As I proceeded to schedule my first solo appointment with you I was able to book my appointment the very next day which once again I knew this had to be more than divine intervention. My first solo appointment I noticed immediate shifts in my life so much I paid for a second solo session. I can't thank you enough for sharing your gifts with the world, your generosity at the end of my second session with a free bonus extra healing but more importantly releasing blocks that have hindered me for years.

You're a true blessing,
L

Thank you so much for the information, Dawn. Today, I woke in a different world with a more positive attitude. You hit the nail on the head with the resisting. Unfortunately, allowing is easier said than done. I allow for infinite possibilities for infinite flow/abundance/happiness in my life every day when I do my chi machine exercise. I have been doing this for several months and I am still waiting. The resistance may be part of the shields I put up years ago when I felt I needed them to protect myself from verbal abuse, etc. Recently, I have been working on lowering those shields even though that leaves me vulnerable again.

I am going to presume my subconscious does not want to let them go. I will work with more of the mp3's that you included in your offer. I know if I am persistent enough, eventually everything will work the way it is supposed to work.

Thank you again for the wonderful session yesterday.

Namaste' and aloha,
D.

Dawn, hi, it's Y****, the last caller from Monday's show. I wanted to write a testimonial and since I couldn't find where to submit it, I thought that I'd just send it to you here: Thank you, thank you, thank you! Those few minutes working with you changed my life completely! Especially in relationships. But most importantly, I finally feel the self-love that I couldn't before. I, for the first time in my life, feel deserving of love.

Thanks again, Much love and blessings to you,
- Y.

Hi Dawn, I was the one who was suicidal the other night when you were on Spaced Out Radio with Elizabeth Anglin. It took a little while, but as the night went on, I progressively felt better, and I wanted to thank you for that.

- L. M.

    HAPPINESS MADE CRYSTAL CLEAR!

I am listening to the Live show right now....and I Feel Fabulous! Thank-You, Thank-You, Thank-You, Dawn Crystal....Many Blessings to you for the Awesome work you do!!!

- D. R.

Dawn, I am in rediscovery. The stranger that was my lost self returned to me by your powerful energy work. I feel clear-headed, balanced, grounded and in total amazement of the self I have to get acquainted with. I am ready for the new world that is coming at us with great speed--and your energy work makes me fearless of whatever the future may hold.

With heartfelt gratitude, and love,
- I.

Hi, Dawn, I had the honor to get selected tonight for you to work with me. I am S., living in ****, NC. I have to admit that when you started in with your sound healing, I said 'What!' I removed my judgment and just went with it. When you selected me for a brief session, I wasn't sure what to expect. While you were working on me, I felt light-headed. After a while, I started to feel lighter and more joyful.

Thank you!
- S.

Hi Darius,

I don't have an intention for this week. Instead, I just wanted to tell you that I bought a package that included a personal session with Dawn Crystal and it is the best thing I have ever done! To put it in a nutshell, I can't even remember why I wanted to work with her. (This is a good thing!). I found a list this morning of things I had wanted to address with her and was shocked that I had felt those things (fear, depression, etc.). **They are just gone**. Anyway, I hope you have her back. She is a true blessing.

By the way, if you use any part of this note for your show, please do not use the name on this email. You can call me Liz from ****** if you need to say anything. (No last name please)

Thanks, LP

Hi, Dawn, thanks so much for the session earlier I feel much lighter already and am looking to clear even more. I'm always so appreciated for your healing. It's really a blessing that you are providing this healing to the world. :)

- A.

I am so Grateful to have had my issues addressed...I slept so good...and I have had a very rough 4 months... Thank You to Dawn Crystal for assisting me....I felt so much calmer after the session...just knowing I was helped in some way

- K.

I appreciate hearing your story that you shared on Lauren's show. I just listened to the replay & the healing I felt was Amazing!!!Your courage to follow your inner guidance is deeply inspiring.

- C. A. H.

Dear Dawn, thank you so very much for the session yesterday. It was right on the money, and I really appreciate everything you did to clear me. I am feeling much lighter, and you really pinpointed some issues for me. I look forward to working with you again.

Take care.
- J.

Hello Dawn, this is J., the first caller on Monday's show. Wow, what an intense session that was!

My body was a rocking and rolling and releasing so much!

I feel like I'm still processing, and I haven't been feeling well (anxious, etc.).

Thank you so much!
- J.

The winter depression has also lessened, and I was able to attend a family function that for years I had not gone to this time of year, and as well, my energy levels are up, which isn't usual for this time of year.

- A.

Hi Dawn, First of all, I have to tell you I absolutely love the work you do and the results I get. I am part of the Learning Strategies Tues. eve. group.

You have been such a blessing in my life. In fact, I listened to last Tuesday's event again early this morning. I know I will sleep well afterward....

C.

Hi Dawn! I wanted to thank you for the healing tonight on Lauren's call! I feel so amazing! I did buy your Higher Self package and I have a session with you this Saturday. I did have a question in the interim; I know you mentioned healing abundance was part of one of the benefits of this package. I was also interested in your Wealth package too.

C.

Hi Dawn,

Wanted to let you know, following my session, this past Sunday, April 15th, I did keep focusing on letting stuff release and integrating higher frequencies. Feelings/emotions did come up and Tuesday evening I got shown and released at a deeper level than ever before an incident with my Dad when I was about 11 yrs that was still impacting me in a very limiting way. I immediately felt more energized, and more capable of 'doing life', creating what I love and desire; shifting from a "I can't" to a "I can" come from/attitude. YAY!!!

And as you said might happen, I did feel some aches/pains in my body following the session, however, that is subsiding. :-)

Thank you sooo much!

And I look forward to our next session at the end of the month!

Love,
L

Hello Dawn,

Delighted to write a testimonial for you:

So many of us work between struggle and hope in our lives. I've been trying to manage anxiety, heal from physical ailments, while also wanting to grow into more abundance and higher energetic integrity. I have found Dawn's voice guidance and acoustic clearings to be enormously helpful and transformative. With dedication, I listen to her modules daily and also regularly journal. In only two weeks, I feel more attuned, expanded and wholly rooted in my own two feet.

Wishing you ever greater circles of influence, and much love,
A

Dawn,

'I've been meaning to send you this testimonial for a few days now but a funny thing has happened. I keep forgetting to write it because I keep forgetting I had any problems. (LOL) I only remembered now because I saw the list I had written before our session that said things like, "I am gripped by fear" or "I feel like my soul has been crushed". I looked at that list this morning and thought, "I was?"... "It did?" I can't even relate to that anymore.

It's taken a minute, but I finally understand why that is. Somehow in that session, it was as if I stepped through a thin veil into a slightly different version of me. It happened so easily and gently that I hardly noticed. The issues associated with the 'other me' have just fallen away and it feels like I have always been the way I am now. I know that sounds totally weird but who cares! I *love* the 'new' me!

I am so incredibly grateful for this transformation and the session. I don't think I have ever felt so 'seen'. To say you have changed my life for the better would be a meager understatement. Thank you, thank you, thank you!!

DP

PS - I also sent a note to ****** to let him know how great it was to work with you.

All the best,
D****

I have purchased three of Dawn's programs and had a session with her. I cannot encourage anyone enough to participate in her wonderful healing love and beautiful vibrations. I felt so much energy and love

                    HAPPINESS MADE CRYSTAL CLEAR!

from Source through her, I was floating. Speaking with her, I felt as I was talking to my long-lost sister. She is a beautiful wonderful, truly loving lady. I am grateful that she shares her beautiful gift with us. I am grateful she has helped me remove my blocks.

Many Blessings,
S.

I have purchased 2 of your packages-Total Body Rejuvenation and Anti-Aging, both from the Eram show, and I think they are brilliant!

I think your work is outstanding and I have done much spiritual and energetic work. Thank you for your pure openness and generosity of spirit!

Much love and light,
M.

Dear Dawn,

Thank you so much for sharing your amazing gifts with me. I am so grateful for your time & effort during my 3 sessions (FHTY - Anti-Aging Package). You are truly one of a kind. Last night's final call session was amazing and releasing the soul (baby) back to Source was so right. He/she would have been attached to me for more than 26 yrs. Finally, now back with Source.

Much Love & with Gratitude,
W

Dawn,

I've tried quite a few different packages from different healers.

Your Anti-aging MP3s are amazing!

When I am listening to them I can feel energy buzzing all around my body, especially at the top of my head.

After listening I feel out of space at the beginning, but later I feel more grounded. I sleep better, I feel better. I feel connected!

Your work is very important and much appreciated.

Much Aloha!

And Blessings!
T

Hello Dawn,

The Anti-aging program works wonders! Mostly all the wrinkles on my face have disappeared and I look ten years younger. I am still working on the perfect weight part, my cravings are less, and I'm eating more fruits and vegetables. My skin is now very soft, and I am glowing. I feel totally different. Thank you Dawn for being who you are today and for helping people, as we all deeply appreciate your work! Thank you so very much!!

C. M.

Dawn,

You have GREATLY helped relief the Pain in my knees and other parts of my Body, with your BODY REJUVENATION package that I purchased via Jazz Up with Judy.

I am SO THANKFUL TO YOU, AND TO SUPREME MOTHER FATHER GOD ALMIGHTY FOR THE WONDERFUL BLESSINGS :)

Looking forward to my 1:1 session with you on NOV 24th

MUCH LOVE & GRATITUDE
and MANY BLESSINGS TO YOU,
N. K.

[Most entries edited for privacy, punctuation, and format.]

Links to Dawn Crystal Recordings

Healing MP3 page
https://dawncrystalmaui.clickfunnels.com/squeeze-page

HEAL ADRENAL FATIQUE & BURNOUT
http://static.wixstatic.com/mp3/14f4a3_cca37fcfbf194e-f08ab3826c85371366.mp3?dn=HEAL+ADRENAL+FATIQUE+&+BURNOUT.mp3

HEALTHY THYROID ACTIVATION
http://static.wixstatic.com/mp3/14f4a3_7d9ba4d1443742e6a3db9639d3f9cd89.mp3?dn=HEALTHY+THYROID+ACTIVATION.mp3

WEIGHT LOSS MADE EASY!!!
http://static.wixstatic.com/mp3/14f4a3_32b6a30cabb44622858a82e25b84ae35.mp3?dn=WEIGHT+LOSS+MADE+EASY%21%21%21.mp3

HAPPY HORMONES ACTIVATION
http://static.wixstatic.com/mp3/14f4a3_7d3083eae81c4130a27bdd54fcfeced8.mp3?dn=HAPPY+HORMONES+ACTIVATION.mp3

HEALTHY GUT ACTIVATION (FREEDOM FROM
DIGESTION ISSUES)
http://static.wixstatic.com/mp3/14f4a3_6575476411644d55926e56
d5a27aa5da.mp3?dn=HEALTHY+GUT+ACTIVATION+%28FREE
DOM+FROM+DIGESTION+ISSUES%29.mp3

ENERGY SYSTEM REBOOT! (RE-ENERGIZE & ALIGN YOUR
ENERGY)
http://static.wixstatic.com/mp3/14f4a3_e8f-
4737fe02c4b878827d567392dbd83.mp3?dn=ENEGY+SYSTEM+R
EBOOT%21%28RE-ENERGIZE+&+ALIGN+YOUR+ENERGY+S
YSTEMS%29.mp3

LIVER CLEANSE & DETOX (DEEP HEALING & RENEWAL)
http://static.wixstatic.com/mp3/14f4a3_115c72702e8c4a5a8351bfb
1fc6d035a.mp3?dn=LIVER+CLEANSE+&+DETOX+%28DEEP+H
EALING+&+RENEWAL%29.mp3

STRESS BE GONE!!! (A DIVINE ENERGY CLEANSING)
http://static.wixstatic.com/mp3/14f4a3_83a2cce86b024f1f9650e58b
9f61a46c.mp3?dn=STRESS+BE+GONE%21%21%21+%28A+DIV
INE+ENERGY+CLEANSING%29.mp3

ALLERGY FREE!!!
http://static.wixstatic.com/mp3/14f4a3_5c7fa5a5bddd4be5a313ad7b
18fa45c4.mp3?dn=ALLERGY+FREE%21%21%21.mp3

CHAKRA CLEARING & BALANCING (FOR PERFECT
HEALTH!)
http://static.wixstatic.com/mp3/14f4a3_ca6abca802e4474084b192a-
c6afff90d.mp3?dn=CHAKRA+CLEARING+&+BALANCING+%2
8FOR+PERFECT+HEALTH%21%29.mp3

HEART LOVE ACTIVATION (OPEN UP TO RECEIVE MORE!!!)
http://static.wixstatic.com/mp3/14f4a3_dc95e9e0dfd94b-fea40f4c96255201db.mp3?dn=HEART+LOVE+ACTIVATION+%28+OPEN+UP+TO+RECEIVE+MORE%21%21%21%29.mp3

KICK-A-HABIT ACTIVATION
http://static.wixstatic.com/mp3/14f4a3_7a1319ba08e84a77b803cf220141b560.mp3?dn=KICK-A-HABIT+ACTIVITATION.mp3

FACE LIFT & EYE LIFT (INCLUDES THE NECK AREA)
http://static.wixstatic.com/mp3/14f4a3_1549829c89234d64917ff300d5b2948b.mp3?dn=FACE+LIFT+&+EYE+LIFT+%28INCLUDES+THE+NECK+AREA%29.mp3

About the Author

Dawn Crystal, an internationally recognized Voice Sound Healer, Body-mind Intuitive, respected Intuitive Life Coach, Soul Reader, Medium, Pain Release Expert and Best-selling Author (*PAIN FREE Made Crystal Clear!*), is known as a **LEADING TRANSFORMATIONAL EXPERT** incorporating ancient wisdom for modern day success.

Dawn is passionate about helping people clear emotional and physical blockages, so they can manifest from their higher selves, step into their full potential, and lead their lives and businesses in ways that align effectively with their souls' purpose.

Dawn helps her clients to release themselves quickly from pain, emotional and physical, and she is an active mentor for entrepreneurs, CEO's, and celebrities, helping everyone! Dawn is the "go-to" person to get out of pain fast, in minutes!

Dawn participates regularly on global teleseminars, radio shows and podcasts. Dawn was recently interviewed by the *Today Show, Dr. Oz, Rachel Ray, The View,* etc. Dawn hosts her own radio show, *Pain Free Fast & Easy!* on the News for the Soul Network. For the past two years she has done a live bi-weekly program at Learning Strategies

Corporation of Minneapolis called, "Sound Healing / Silent Clearing."

Dawn's unique sound healing CD has been purchased by clients around the globe, and she is available on both phone and Skype, as well as for teleseminars.

Dawn lives a peaceful life on Maui, along with her adorable dog, Hoku.

Dawn recently published two books in this series, *PAIN FREE Made Crystal Clear* and *FEAR FREE Made Crystal Clear*, both published by Outskirts Press, available in paperback and ebook formats from Outskirts and from Amazon (amazon.com) and Barnes & Noble (bn. com).

"I wouldn't change anything about my life; it's a gift," Dawn affirms, and she transmits this inner strength to those she works with, giving them a grounding, a stable psychological place abounding with safety and love.

"I wouldn't do it over again, but I am glad where I ended up."

To see a ten-minute interview video with Dawn Crystal, go to

https://tinyurl.com/ybg3osgp.

Review Happiness?

Reviews on sites such as amazon.com help connect readers and authors. We would appreciate it if you would write a review, even a short one.